SpringerBriefs in Computer Science

Series editors

Stan Zdonik, Brown University, Providence, USA
Shashi Shekhar, University of Minnesota, Minneapolis, USA
Jonathan Katz, University of Maryland, College Park, USA
Xindong Wu, University of Vermont, Burlington, USA
Lakhmi C. Jain, University of South Australia, Adelaide, Australia
David Padua, University of Illinois Urbana-Champaign, Urbana, USA
Xuemin (Sherman) Shen, University of Waterloo, Waterloo, Canada
Borko Furht, Florida Atlantic University, Boca Raton, USA
V.S. Subrahmanian, University of Maryland, College Park, USA
Martial Hebert, Carnegie Mellon University, Pittsburgh, USA
Katsushi Ikeuchi, University of Tokyo, Tokyo, Japan
Bruno Siciliano, Università di Napoli Federico II, Napoli, Italy
Sushil Jajodia, George Mason University, Fairfax, USA
Newton Lee, Newton Lee Laboratories, Tujunga, USA

More information about this series at http://www.springer.com/series/10028

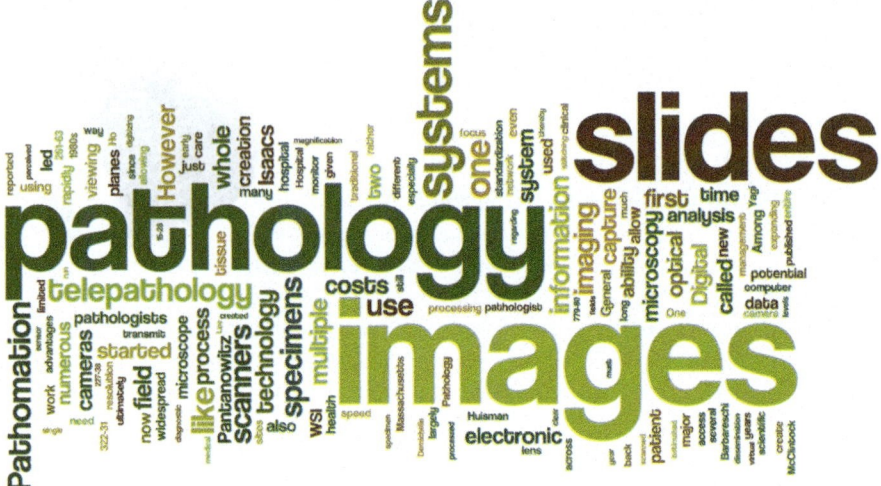

Yves Sucaet · Wim Waelput

Digital Pathology

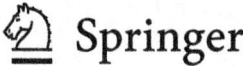 Springer

Yves Sucaet
Wim Waelput
Pathomation
Berchem
Belgium

ISSN 2191-5768   ISSN 2191-5776   (electronic)
ISBN 978-3-319-08779-5   ISBN 978-3-319-08780-1   (eBook)
DOI 10.1007/978-3-319-08780-1

Library of Congress Control Number: 2014943501

Springer Cham Heidelberg New York Dordrecht London

© The Author(s) 2014
This work is subject to copyright. All rights are reserved by the Publisher, whether the whole or part of the material is concerned, specifically the rights of translation, reprinting, reuse of illustrations, recitation, broadcasting, reproduction on microfilms or in any other physical way, and transmission or information storage and retrieval, electronic adaptation, computer software, or by similar or dissimilar methodology now known or hereafter developed. Exempted from this legal reservation are brief excerpts in connection with reviews or scholarly analysis or material supplied specifically for the purpose of being entered and executed on a computer system, for exclusive use by the purchaser of the work. Duplication of this publication or parts thereof is permitted only under the provisions of the Copyright Law of the Publisher's location, in its current version, and permission for use must always be obtained from Springer. Permissions for use may be obtained through RightsLink at the Copyright Clearance Center. Violations are liable to prosecution under the respective Copyright Law.
The use of general descriptive names, registered names, trademarks, service marks, etc. in this publication does not imply, even in the absence of a specific statement, that such names are exempt from the relevant protective laws and regulations and therefore free for general use.
While the advice and information in this book are believed to be true and accurate at the date of publication, neither the authors nor the editors nor the publisher can accept any legal responsibility for any errors or omissions that may be made. The publisher makes no warranty, express or implied, with respect to the material contained herein.

Printed on acid-free paper

Springer is part of Springer Science+Business Media (www.springer.com)

To Lilly and Lucas

Preface

Dr. Sucaet holds a Ph.D. in Bioinformatics from Iowa State University. His research background is in systems and network biology. He is a co-founder of Pathomation and currently fulfills the role of Chief Technology Officer. Before that, he was at HistoGeneX in the function of Section Head, Data Management and Bioinformatics, where he met Dr. Waelput. They decided to combine their expertise and have been promoting the use of digital pathology ever since.

Dr. Waelput is an M.D. and certified pathologist, currently employed as a senior staff member at the University Hospital of Brussels (UZ-Brussels). He is also a consulting (pharma-)pathologist at HistoGeneX and a co-founder of Pathomation. Dr. Waelput has been involved in research on protein–protein interactions and signal transduction within the Department of Medical Protein Research at the Flemish Institute for Biotechnology (VIB—Vlaams Instituut voor Biotechnologie). He obtained his Ph.D. from the University of Ghent.

Pathomation is a young innovative company founded in 2012. The company was created by two pathologists and a bioinformatician. Located in Berchem, Belgium, the company strives to offer the most comprehensive software platform for digital pathology possible. The focus is on integration, scalability, and user-friendliness. Pathomation implements digital pathology in a variety of use cases and scenarios. Truly vendor-independent digital pathology solutions are hard to come by. Platforms that claim to be vendor-independent are difficult to adapt to specific circumstances. Interoperability, which is taken for granted in wet lab conditions (e.g., a sample is sectioned on a Leica microtome, stained on a Dako autostainer, and studied under an Olympus microscope), is often lacking when moving to digital pathology. Therefore, Pathomation develops software for pathologists, designed by pathologists. Its PathoCore software can read most proprietary vendor formats, so the company is not tied to any technology and can offer objective guidance. PathoCore is central to a complete software platform. In addition, other applications are available, including viewers and host application plug-ins. Because of this component-based architecture, Pathomation is ideally placed to take digital pathology information (including augmented datasets like on-slide annotations and captured form-data) and deliver it to any target environment or device.

This work would not have been possible without the valuable input of several others. We would like to thank, in alphabetical order:

David Ameisen
Essam E. Ayad
Peter Lang
Zev Leifer
Mathieu Malaterre
Koen Marien
Agelos Pappas
Yukako Yagi

And a special thank you to Simon Rees and Wayne Wheeler of Springer for guiding us through the publishing process.

Contents

1 **Digital Pathology's Past to Present** 1
   1.1 Introduction 1
   1.2 Beginnings and Evolution 3
       1.2.1 Reaching Out: Telepathology Networks 4
       1.2.2 Digital Pathology and Whole Slide Imaging 5
       1.2.3 Differences with Radiology 7
   1.3 Successes and Challenges 8
   1.4 Digital Pathology Today...................................... 9
   1.5 Preliminary Conclusions 10
   References... 10

2 **Hardware and Software** 15
   2.1 How Are Digital Pathology Images "Captured"?................. 15
   2.2 How Do Slide Scanners Work? 17
   2.3 Virtual Slide Formats 20
       2.3.1 How Are WSI Data Organized?........................ 20
       2.3.2 The Pyramidal Format 20
       2.3.3 Tiles 20
       2.3.4 Color Spaces... 21
       2.3.5 Compression Schemes 22
   2.4 Vendor-Specific File Format Implementations................... 22
       2.4.1 TIFF-Based Formats................................. 22
       2.4.2 Other Format Types 25
       2.4.3 The Role of DICOM................................. 27
   2.5 Bits, Bytes, and Wires 27
   References... 28

3 **Applications** 31
   3.1 Education 31
   3.2 Remote Consultations and Second Opinions.................... 33
   3.3 Tumor Boards and Pathology Reviews 34

3.4	Biobanking and Collection Hosting	35
3.5	Primary Diagnosis	38
	3.5.1 In the USA: The Role of the FDA	38
	3.5.2 Throughout the Rest of the World	39
3.6	Birds of a Feather	40
References		40

4 Image Analysis 43
    4.1 Current Technology and Challenges 43
    4.2 Current State of Digital Pathology and WSI Analysis 48
    4.3 Toward In Silico Pathology 50
    References 50

5 Use Cases 57
    5.1 Diagnosis and Staging of Disease 57
        5.1.1 Biomarkers 57
        5.1.2 Cytology 60
    5.2 Digital Pathology as a Teaching Tool 62
        5.2.1 New York College of Podiatric Medicine 62
        5.2.2 Universal Education 63
    5.3 Telepathology in Developing Countries 64
        5.3.1 E-Education and Telepathology in Egypt 65
        5.3.2 Heavy Lifting in Port-au-Prince, Haiti 66
    5.4 Quality Control and Assurance 67
    5.5 Tremendous Potential 68
    References 69

6 A Bright Future 71
    6.1 The 5 %/$2.4 Billion Challenge 71
    6.2 New Frontiers 72
        6.2.1 Medical Systems Biology 72
        6.2.2 Three-Dimensional WSI 73
        6.2.3 Spectral Imaging 74
        6.2.4 Extending the Pathology Value Chain, Upstream,
                and Downstream 75
    6.3 Hope for the Third World 76
    6.4 Digital Pathology DIY 77
    6.5 Final Conclusions 78
    6.6 Learn More About Digital Pathology 78
    References 79

Retraction Note: Hardware and Software E1

About the Authors 81

Index 83

Chapter 1
Digital Pathology's Past to Present

Abstract Digital pathology is a rapidly growing field that did not even exist 20 years ago. However, in some ways, its origins date back to the earliest attempts at telepathology back in the 1960s. This chapter provides a brief historical perspective on how digital pathology came to be. It answers questions like why does it exist and what need does it fulfill? It also provides a brief summary of current applications and the challenges ahead; explains why we believe digital pathology is rapidly coming of age; and describes the converging factors that lead us to this conclusion.

Keywords Digital pathology · Digital pathology history · Telepathology · Informatics · Whole slide imaging · Pathology cockpit · Pathology dashboard · WSI · DP

1.1 Introduction

One of the world's most renowned and successful inventors, the late Charles Franklin Kettering (1876–1958), also was a very gifted man of words. Among his most famous lines are: "Our imagination is the only limit to what we can hope to have in the future" and "People are very open-minded about new things—as long as they're exactly like the old ones." These two statements encapsulate the struggles that exist with any novel idea, and certainly with any new field, whether that field is in engineering, science, art, or medicine.

Among the very newest of fields in medicine is the field of digital pathology which, as a distinct entity, only started to be mentioned in published, peer-reviewed scientific journals in the year 2000 [1–3], though its roots reach at least into the 1990s [4] and perhaps even further. Initially, relatively little was written about digital pathology; but this has changed dramatically, especially over the last 5 years. In fact, in a recent (April 2014) search for "digital pathology" (with two quotation marks to specifically isolate this term), only 188 relevant abstracts were identified, of which 164 (87 %) had been published from 2009 onward.

Digital pathology, in its simplest form, is the conversion of the optical image of a classic pathologic slide into a digital image that can then be uploaded onto a computer for viewing; and this is very much what it started out to be. Single, two-dimensional virtual slides, followed by virtual cases involving several slides [1–3, 5] were the first forays into the field of digital pathology. Since then, however, the concept and functionality of digital pathology has grown exponentially, so that a more accurate current definition would be that it is the field of anatomic and microanatomic pathology information systems. These systems allow not only for the visualization of specimens in digital form, but also for the complete electronic management of two- and three-dimensional specimens, allowing for their real-time evaluation, comparison, two- to three-dimensional reconstruction, archiving, dissemination for widespread viewing and consultation, compilation with other patient data, data mining, and use for education, clinical diagnosis and patient management, research, and the development of artificial intelligence tools [6–9], and this may still only be scratching the surface.

Early pioneers in the field foresaw numerous obstacles that would be faced in the creation of useable interconnected digital pathology systems, but believed that they were both surmountable and worth overcoming [1, 3, 5, 10]. Among the many readily perceived additional advantages of digital over standard pathology practices included and continue to include the relative permanence of digital files versus glass slides; the ability to access past specimens from the same or some other patient without having to hunt down previous slides and possibly restain them; the potential to compare multiple slides simultaneously on the same monitor screen (e.g., to put normal tissue "control" slides and "pathology" slides side by side); the ability to draft reports or comments in the same window; the ability to annotate (circle, label, add arrows, etc.); the tremendous potential for research and teaching; the relative ease of viewing one or many slides on a monitor with mouse-click control of magnitude and orientation versus the eye-exhausting process of peering through a microscope lens at one slide at a time; and, perhaps most of all, the ability to transmit digital images over distances to allow for the creation of an integrated network of pathologists who could now work together in multiple different contexts to enhance patient care [1, 5, 11] (Fig. 1.1).

As will be discussed in the following pages, this broad range of potential uses for digital pathology has led both to its rapidly expanding use across an even broader range of indications, and to an ever-growing requirement for expanded, advanced, and enhanced technology to support all these functions. This technology started with a desire to transmit (digital) images of pathology slides to distant sites, primarily for the purposes of obtaining the opinions of off-site pathologists, a process which has been called *telepathology*.

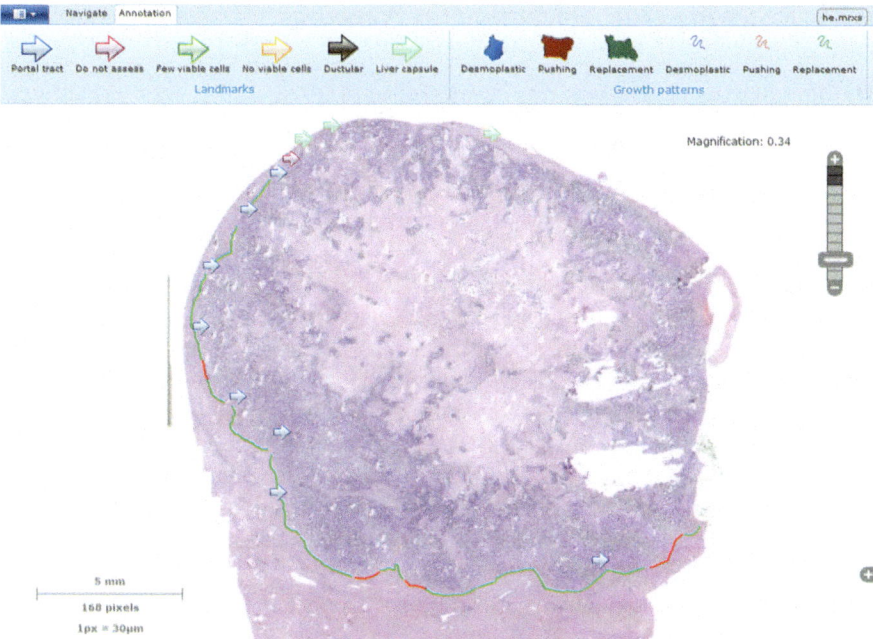

Fig. 1.1 An example of how our own in-house developed viewer software can be used to annotate different features on a digital slide

1.2 Beginnings and Evolution

On February 9, 2009, United States President Barack Obama said: "We have the most inefficient health care system imaginable. We're still using paper. Nurses can't read the prescriptions that doctors have written out. Why wouldn't we want to put that on an electronic medical record that will reduce error rates, reduce our long-term costs of health care, and create jobs right now?" [12].

With that statement and a subsequent federal economic stimulus package called the American Recovery and Reinvestment Act (ARRA) of 2009 that President Obama signed into law on February 17, 2009, Health Information Technology (HIT) achieved a new level of prominence in the USA. But the move toward creating a system of electronic records that would allow for the paperless storage and transmission of health information started decades before this, with the development of, albeit very limited, systems to transmit information between sites and centers using the primitive computer technology of the day. It progressed as computer technology progressed, leading first to networks that would allow for the sharing of information between multiple sites, but ultimately progressing to all-encompassing health information systems capable of infinitely more.

1.2.1 Reaching Out: Telepathology Networks

The first digital camera was not developed until 1975, and it was virtually two decades later before they started to gain widespread commercial popularity [13]. However, when black and white microscopy (digital) images were transmitted from Boston's Logan Airport to Massachusetts General Hospital way back in 1968 [14], it was a huge step toward recognizing one of the primary advantages of such technology: the ability to convert pathology slides into (digital) images that could then be transmitted across distances. Transmitting these microscopy images only was feasible because a rudimentary laboratory information system, called the Massachusetts General Hospital Utility Multi-programming System (MUMPS), had been created as a collaboration between Massachusetts General Hospital and a company called Bolt Beranek Newman [15]. At about the same time, General Electric announced their intentions to create a commercially available hospital information system through a subsidiary called MediNet. However, given perceived astronomical costs and complexities, this plan ultimately was abandoned [16]. Further attempts to create such systems failed repeatedly throughout much of the 1970s, largely because programming tools and computer technology were inadequate [17]. Among the various problems encountered was that, despite enormous sizes relative to modern-day computers, systems generally lacked the computing power to handle any more than a single user or interface at a given time. It was not until the 1980s that technology companies such as Intel and IBM started to rapidly enhance their ability to construct semiconductors, resulting in what was quickly termed *Moore's Law*: the doubling of available computing power every one to 2 years. Meanwhile, standardized, easy-to-use, increasingly powerful, and highly portable programming languages emerged, such as Pascal and C/C+; and Intel's x86 instruction set architecture, initially released with the Intel 8086 CPU in 1978 to increase the unit's memory capacity from 8 to 16 bits, rose to prominence [18]. This, in turn, led to the creation of more powerful and much more user-friendly relational database management systems, and their eventual integration into workplaces that included clinical laboratories. Ultimately, however, it was creation of the World Wide Web in the 1990s that led to the widespread development and use of data transmission systems that now comprise one of the cornerstones of digital pathology, overcoming the greatest challenge that was faced with the first systems. Transmitting pathology data from one laboratory to a distant site was becoming not only feasible, but almost instantaneous.

Informatics has been defined as "the discipline focused on the acquisition, storage, and use of information in a specific setting or domain [12]." Discussion about creating a digital informatics environment began as early as the late 1970s and early 1980s, but among radiologists rather than pathologists [19, 20]. It was not until in the mid- to late 1980s that the term *telepathology*, which Weinstein et al. [21, 22] defined as "the practice of pathology over a long distance," made its first appearance in the scientific literature. Components of the first telepathology systems included a remote-controlled light microscope attached to a

1.2 Beginnings and Evolution

high-resolution video camera; a pathologist workstation that incorporated controls for manipulating the microscope; a high-resolution video monitor; and some form of telecommunications linkage [21]. The first published report of a telepathology network linking multiple facilities was by Weinstein et al. [23], who described their international pathology network linking pathology services across four cities in Arizona and two international sites: one in China and the other in Mexico. By the mid-1990s, telepathology was gaining momentum. But it was not until the commercial availability of digital cameras and scanners, followed by their integration into medical practice and ultimate linkage to the World Wide Web, that the true potential of telepathology took a giant leap forward [24], ultimately allowing for the creation of digitally based pathology service networks far grander than anything initially proposed or likely even conceived by Weinstein or anyone else in the mid-1990s [14, 21–23, 25, 26].

1.2.2 Digital Pathology and Whole Slide Imaging

With its emergence in the twenty-first century, digital pathology has represented a fundamental change in the way pathological specimens are viewed. Instead of viewing glass slides or other specimens through a microscope, such specimens can now be examined through a digital monitor. The most essential element of this process is a device to digitally capture images (image digitization). To date, such devices include digital cameras and digital scanners.

Digital cameras work by recording (optical) images not on film, as classic cameras do, but on electronic image sensors. These electronic sensors, in turn, generate electronic signals that are converted into long digital sequences (of "1"s and "0"s). By sampling, which involves digitizing the coordinate values, and by quantization, which is digitizing the amplitude values, we obtain a digital image of the optical image. In truth, there are actually four principle images: (1) There is the *optical image*, which is created by the lens system; (2) There is the *digital image*, which is created by digitizing the optical image; (3) There is the *displayed image*, which is the digital image converted; and (4) There is the *continuous image*, which is its mathematical representation.

To function, each digital camera contains a built-in microcomputer, to which images are saved for later editing, viewing, and transfer to other devices. Like digital cameras, digital slide scanners contain electronic image sensors that generate electronic signals; but, unlike cameras, slide scanners allow for the capture of multiple images during movement of the sensor, without moving the object of interest. And where cameras must be placed on top of a microscope, scanners completely bypass the need for a camera (which is built into the scanner in that case).

Low- to medium-resolution scanners were being used commercially and in clinical settings long before digital cameras ever gained popularity. In the clinical setting, their first use was as early as the 1980s. However, such use was only for single-function purposes like the DNA sequencing of gel auto-radiographs, measuring immunofluorescence in stained cells, quantifying immunoblots, and copying figures and other images, like slides, for scientific publications [27–31]. These early scanners lacked both the resolution and functionality of twenty-first-century scanners. To be functional for digital pathology, both functions needed to undergo significant enhancements.

Digital pathology images must have sufficient contrast in order to visualize individual cells and their characteristics. As with digital photography, image contrast is determined by the optical components (the lens) and the image sensor: the smaller the pixel spacing in the sensor and the better the resolution of the lens, the more finely resolved the optical image can be captured without sampling distortion (also called *pixelation or under-sampling*). However, achieving higher-contrast images comes with its own challenges and costs, like greater memory requirements and higher bandwidth capacity to capture, upload, and transmit these digital optical images of adequate resolution.

One of the many advances in digital pathology that has occurred over time relates to the creation of the pathologist's new work station, which has been called a *digital cockpit* or *digital dashboard* [32], so that it enhances each pathologist's ability to access, visualize, interpret, and share digital pathology images and thereby utilize digital informatics systems effectively and efficiently. One major problem with dashboards, and in fact with most components of telepathology and digital pathology systems, has been their lack of standardization.

Another major accomplishment that had its origins with seminal work that was reported by Ferreira et al. [4], but which truly only started to be used clinically in the new millennium [33], has been the evolution from capturing individual microscopy fields for review to whole slide imaging (WSI). This process requires specialized scanners that are both high-resolution and high-speed and that can digitize images across large arrays and combine these images, through a process called *stitching*, into even larger arrays [34–36]. As such, not just certain fields of a slide, but entire slides can be visualized. Moreover, they can be scanned at multiple levels of magnification and in all three planes (x, y, and z) [14]. One major advantage of stitching numerous images together rather than trying to capture entire slides at once relates to the former allowing for images to be brought into focus and then captured at higher levels of magnification, rather than having to capture the entire slide at lower magnification and later enlarge it, thereby tampering with focus and losing resolution. However, stitching creates its own complications, like ensuring that the lighting, focus, and coloring of each of the partial images match, especially since the topology of the specimen may vary from one part of the specimen to another. This has led to numerous process refinements, like shading and lighting normalization, auto-focusing, and independent dual-sensor scanning that allows for image acquisition and focusing to be performed sequentially, rather than in the same step [37, 38].

Scanning at different levels (i.e., different focal planes) must be distinguished from zooming in, which refers to magnification within a single plane, both of which are useful, but for different reasons. Whereas magnification allows for closer inspection and better detection of smaller structures, the ability to scan

1.2 Beginnings and Evolution

tissues at different levels and in all three planes has led to the generation of three-dimensional image reproductions of original tissue, which is achieved by scanning multiple focal planes into images and then stacking them, a process that is invaluable for the evaluation of cytological specimens, frozen sections, and other thick specimens where the pathologist needs to assess cellular architecture in multiple planes. In this way, entire tissue sections can be visualized [39–42]. Thick specimens can not only be scanned throughout, but the focal plane can be rotated in any direction. In addition, as will be elaborated further in Chap. 4, stains can be both detected and quantified [43, 44]. This is accomplished using recent innovations like *automated (histopathology) pattern recognition* [45]; color enhancement, and standardization techniques [46–48], as well as *color content analysis* that allows for the detection and quantification of histochemical stains [49]; and *image microarrays* (IMA) and *multiplexed biomarker testing* so that several tissue characteristics, biomarkers, or stains can be sought and detected on the same slide, thereby replacing the tedious-to-make and difficult-to-maintain cell and tissue (paraffin) blocks of traditional microscopy [50, 51].

Despite all these functions, systems have become faster and now have capacities to multitask. Not just one slide, but numerous slides or tissue specimens, captured in many different focal planes, can be imaged. Detecting or quantifying several different cellular characteristics, like the uptake of fluorescent stain, can be processed at the same time. In addition, data can be extracted from the images and tested, using various algorithms that allow for the automatic detection and characterization of, as an example, cancerous cells [52]. Automated image analysis of routine histological sections is now being used to detect and quantify the expression of human epidermal growth factor receptor (HER-2) in breast cancer, since over-expression is associated with an increased risk of recurrence and poor outcomes [53]. It also predicts responsiveness to trastuzumab, a monoclonal antibody that targets the HER2/neu receptor [53].

1.2.3 Differences with Radiology

Notice how we call it "radiology," and not "digital radiology." That is because radiology already is digital. We take it for granted, so we omit the "digital" adjective. We estimate that pathology is about 10 years behind radiology in terms of digitization. It is tempting therefore to think that solutions devised for radiology can be replicated or even reused for pathology.

However, it is important to recognize that pathology is fundamentally different from radiology, and there are reasons why digital pathology lags behind. First, the source material is different: radiology usually works with live specimens (patients), whereby pathology usually concerns specimen samples (biopsies, cytologies). Protocols also are fundamentally different in pathology, whereby additional stains often are requested by the pathologist, based on observations made in the original H&E stained slide. This constant interchange between digital observations and wet laboratory techniques poses new challenges for laboratory information systems, which is just one reason RIS-software (Radiology Information System) is not a good fit for today's pathology departments (and therefore cannot be easily ported either).

Digital pathology has a number of intrinsic advantages as well. The whole slide images are representations of physical (stained) microscopy slides, which are archived by most hospitals. This means that in the simple case where an image is unfocused, it suffices often to simply rescan the original slide. This is not nearly so easy in radiology, where a patient has to be contacted and rescheduled.

Finally, radiology has the technical advantage of only having to be concerned with grayscale images. This means that calibration standards are available for both scanners and display devices [such as grayscale standard display function (GSDF)]. This sets a data representation standard for a wide array of imaging data. Chromogenic stains in digital pathology are by definition in color. Work on a standard representation of color has only just gotten underway [48, 54]. Also, all of these efforts are complicated by the fact that staining intensities themselves are difficult to replicate across different laboratories and time periods (e.g., "how 'pink and purple' must an HE-stain be to be considered accurate?").

1.3 Successes and Challenges

Two questions arise: "Can such systems accurately identify pathology?" and "Are pathologists actually using such systems in numbers or to an extent that justifies their continued development?" Several studies have been published comparing traditional light microscopy with WSI, as will be discussed in detail in Chap. 4, where we will focus on the use of digital pathology systems not just for image capture and viewing, but automatic image analysis. Although it is beyond the scope of this chapter to review all of the scientific evidence justifying the use of digital scanning/WSI in pathology, what is clear is that many of the obstacles initially envisioned have been addressed. As such, the value and potential uses of digital pathology are expanding exponentially, in parallel with advances in technology [6, 14, 25, 36, 40, 55].

This being said, data on how much digital pathology actually is being utilized are scant. In 2005, Dennis et al. [56] published the results of their survey of consultant histopathologists randomly selected from the membership of the Royal College of Pathologists in the United Kingdom. Among the 47 % who responded, 64 % reported having a digital camera mounted on their microscope; however, only 12 % had any sort of telepathology equipment and only 24 % had ever used telepathology in a diagnostic situation. Moreover, 59 % reported having received no training in digital imaging. In another study assessing its use in the year 2010 by a single academic pathology group that generates roughly 380,000 slides per year, only 2.7 % of all slides were scanned [57]. However, value-added analysis revealed numerous significant benefits of WSI over standard practices, in terms of patient care, educational programs, and research. Five specific advantages related to patient care were image versus slide availability, time to access, portability, and permanence, as well as production of a substrate for digital image analysis. Areas in which WSI was perceived to be of particular value were when slides are sent or received from other facilities, when slides are destroyed by ancillary testing, when slides are used in medicolegal cases, and when slides specifically warrant digital image analysis [57]. Areas in which WSI was not perceived to be advantageous, at that time, largely related to costs and the lack of any evidence suggesting that digital pathology enhances diagnostic accuracy despite these increased costs. For example, whereas overnight shipping of slides at a given hospital was estimated at just $4,000 annually, the costs of a new 5-slide scanner was estimated at $135,000–160,000 [57].

In Japan, the results of a survey conducted in 2008 and 2009 revealed still limited but rapidly expanding use of digital pathology, including its incorporation into the national hospital information system in 2006 [58]. However, it still was being used uncommonly for diagnostic consultation purposes, largely due to limited access to visual slide systems.

Concerns that drive low utilization rates also include doubts about the overall quality of images [59]; reservations about user experience [59]; the monetary costs of high-speed, high-capacity slide scanners, which typically run between $100,000 and $250,000 [59] with operating costs that can run up to $650,000 annually [59]; and concerns that digital pathology will not only replace standard pathology techniques, but pathologists themselves [60, 61].

1.4 Digital Pathology Today

Two further, major obstacles that remain in the way of digital pathology's widespread adoption are the lack of standardization and issues regarding workload and speed. Numerous component processes are involved in the processing of each whole slide image, starting with image capture and analysis, but progressing through to archiving, retrieval, and dissemination. In light of this, national and international efforts are being undertaken to standardize each stage, orchestrated by organizations like the Digital Pathology Association, International Academy of Digital Pathology, the College of American Pathologists' Diagnostic Intelligence and Health Information (DIHIT) Committee, and EURO-TELEPATH, the primary telepathology network in Europe [6, 62–64].

The second major obstacle relates to the volume of slides that would need to be processed for WSI to largely replace traditional microscopy, and the speed and efficiency with which this can be achieved. Some pathology laboratories process tremendous volumes of slides; for example, Isaacs et al. [57] reported that their facility processed roughly 15,000 slides daily. Meanwhile, at Massachusetts General Hospital, given average scan times per image of 60–90 s, McClintock et al. [65] estimated that the hospital would need not just one, but several additional WSI robots beyond the one they already possessed for its digital pathology system to keep up with demands, if WSI was indeed to replace traditional microscopy. This concern regarding image-processing speed has led to a proliferation of WSI management systems designed to enhance the capture, storage, retrieval, and dissemination of virtual slides and specimens [32, 66–68]; though, as noted above, they have yet to be standardized.

As will be expanded upon in Chaps. 3 and 5, one area in which digital pathology is receiving widespread acceptance is as an educational tool [7, 36, 58, 64, 69, 70]. Its advantages in terms of creating a permanent, easily accessible, and readily transferrable system of pathology slide and specimen archiving are also clear. Whether the full adoption of WSI occurs within the next 5–15 years [65], as some have suggested, or indeed ever remains to be seen. What is clear is that it is a rapidly expanding and evolving tool in the field of pathology. There is full reason to believe that what we see of WSI today is merely scratching the surface.

1.5 Preliminary Conclusions

Though the term *digital pathology* did not appear in the medical literature until roughly 2000, its origins reach back further, starting with the very first transfer of black and white microscopy slides from an airport to a hospital in 1968. However, it has been since 2000, and especially over the last half decade that the field has started to experience exponential growth. Starting with simple single images, current scanners have evolved to be able to take dozens of images simultaneously in multiple planes, to stack them to create 3-D tissue reproductions, and to analyze them with advanced algorithms, allowing for the automated diagnoses and differentiation of numerous pathological conditions. Challenges remain, however, especially since their use continues to be limited to a minority of pathologists, and because of concerns regarding processing speed, the standardization of the numerous processing steps, and how WSI ultimately will influence careers in pathology. Much work must be done and is being done to allay these concerns.

References

1. Barbareschi, M., Demichelis, F., Forti, S., Dalla Palma, P.: Digital pathology: science fiction? Int. J. Surg. Pathol. **8**, 261–263 (2000)
2. Danielsen, H.E., Kildal, W., Sudbo, J.: Digital image analysis in pathology—exemplified in prostatic cancer. Tidsskr Nor Laegeforen. **120**, 479–488 (2000). Article in Norwegian
3. Saltz, J.H.: Digital pathology—the big picture. Hum. Pathol. **31**, 779–780 (2000)
4. Ferreira, R., Moon, B., Humphries, J. et al. The virtual microscope. In: Proceedings of AMIA Annual Fall Symposium, 1997, pp. 449–453
5. Demichelis, F., Barbareschi, M., Dalla Palma, P., Forti, S.: The virtual case: a new method to completely digitize cytological and histological slides. Virchows. Arch. **441**, 159–164 (2002)
6. Rojo, M.G.: State of the art and trends for digital pathology. Stud. Health Technol. Inform. **179**, 15–28 (2012)

References

7. Huisman, A.: Digital pathology for education. Stud. Health Technol. Inform. **179**, 68–71 (2012)
8. Slodowska, J., Garcia-Rojo, M.: Digital pathology in personalized cancer therapy. Stud. Health Technol. Inform. **179**, 143–154 (2012)
9. Song, Y., Treanor, D., Bulpitt, A.J., Magee, D.R.: 3D reconstruction of multiple stained histology images. J. Pathol. Inform. **4**, S7 (2013)
10. Wells, C.A., Sowter, C.: Telepathology: a diagnostic tool for the millennium? J Pathol. **191**, 1–7 (2000)
11. Coleman, R.: Can histology and pathology be taught without microscopes? The advantages and disadvantages of virtual histology. Acta Histochem. **111**, 1–4 (2009)
12. Hersh, W.: A stimulus to define informatics and health information technology. BMC Med. Inform. Decis. Mak. **9**, 24 (2009)
13. Prakel, D.: The Visual Dictionary of Photography, p. 91. AVA Publishing, New York (2009)
14. Pantanowitz, L.: Digital images and the future of digital pathology. J. Pathol. Inform. **10**, 1 (2010)
15. Barnett, G.O., Castleman, P.A.: A time-sharing computer system for patient-care activities. Comput. Biomed. Res. **1**, 41–51 (1967)
16. Barnett, G.O.: History of the development of medical information at the Laboratory of Computer Science at Massachusetts General Hospital. In: Blum, B.I., Duncan, K. (eds.) In A History of Medical Informatics, pp. 141–153. AMC Press, New York (1990)
17. Park, S.L., Pantanowitz, L., Sharma, G., Parwani, A.V.: Anatomic pathology laboratory information systems: a review. Adv. Anat. Pathol. **19**, 81–96 (2012)
18. Teorey, T.J., Lightstone, S.S., Nadeau, T., et al.: Database Modeling and Design: Logical Design, 5th edn. Morgan Kaufmann Publishers, Waltham (2011)
19. Lemke, H.U.: A network of medical work stations for integrated word and picture communication in clinical medicine. Technical Report. Berlin, Technical University (1979)
20. Capp, M.P., Nudelman, S.: Photoelectronic radiology department. Proc. SPIE **314**, 2–8 (1981)
21. Weinstein, R.S., Bloom, K.J., Rozek, L.S.: Telepathology and the networking of pathology diagnostic services. Arch. Pathol. Lab. Med. **111**, 646–652 (1987)
22. Weinstein, R.S.: Prospects for telepathology. Hum. Pathol. **17**, 433–434 (1986)
23. Weinstein, R.S., Bhattacharyya, A.K., Yu, Y.P., et al.: Pathology consultation services via the Arizona-International Telemedicine Network. Arch. Anat. Cytol. Pathol. **43**, 219–226 (1995)
24. Furness, P.N.: The use of digital images in pathology. J. Pathol. **183**, 253–263 (1997)
25. Pantanowicz, L., Szymas, J., Yagi, Y., and Wilbur, D. Whole slide imaging for educational purposes. J. Pathol. Inform., vol **3**. (2012)
26. Williams, S., Henricks, W.H., Becich, M.J., Toscano, M., Carter, A.B.: Telepathology for patient care: what am I getting myself into? Adv. Anat. Pathol. **17**, 130–149 (2010)
27. Elder, J.K., Green, D.K., Southern, E.M.: Automatic reading of DNA sequencing gel autoradiographs using a large format digital scanner. Nucleic Acids Res. **14**, 417–424 (1986)
28. Jaggi, B., Poon, S.S., MacAulay, C., Palcic, B.: Imaging system for morphometric assessment of absorption or fluorescence in stained cells. Cytometry **9**, 566–572 (1988)
29. Montague, P.R., Meyer, M., Folberg, R.: Technique for the digital imaging of histopathologic preparations of eyes for research and publication. Ophthalmology **102**, 1248–1251 (1995)
30. Schenk, M.P., Manning, R.J., Paalman, M.H.: Going digital: image preparation for biomedical publishing. Anat. Rec. **257**, 128–136 (1999)
31. Velleman, S.G.: Quantifying immunoblots with a digital scanner. Biotechniques **18**, 1056–1058 (1995)
32. Krupinski, E.A.: Optimizing the pathology workstation "cockpit": challenges and solutions. J. Pathol. Inform. **1**, 19 (2010)
33. Judkins, A.R.: Digital pathology: a tool for 21st century neuropathology. Brain Pathol. **19**, 305 (2009)
34. Silage, D.A., Gil, J.: Digital image tiles: a method for the processing of large sections. J. Microsc. **138**, 221–227 (1985)
35. Westerkamp, D., Gahm, T.: Non-distorted assemblage of the digital images of adjacent fields in histological sections. Anal. Cell Pathol. **5**, 235–247 (1993)

36. Wilbur, D.C.: Digital cytology: current state of the art and prospects for the future. Acta Cytol. **55**, 227–238 (2011)
37. McKay, R.R., Baxi, V.A., Montalto, M.C.: The accuracy of dynamic predictive autofocusing for whole slide imaging. J. Pathol. Inform. **2**, 38 (2011)
38. Montalto, M.C., McKay, R.R., Filkins, R.J.: Autofocus methods of whole slide imaging systems and the introduction of a second-generation independent dual sensor scanning method. J. Pathol. Inform. **2**, 44 (2011)
39. CFR—Code of Federal Regulations Title 21. U.S. Food and Drug Administration 2014
40. Al-Janabi, S., Huisman, A., Van Diest, P.J.: Digital pathology: current status and future perspectives. Histopathology **61**, 1–9 (2012)
41. Chantrain, C.F., DeClerck, Y.A., Groshen, S., McNamara, G.: Computerized quantification of tissue vascularization using high-resolution slide scanning of whole tumor sections. J. Histochem. Cytochem. **51**, 151–158 (2003)
42. Kalinski, T., Zwonitzer, R., Sel, S., et al.: Virtual 3D microscopy using multiplane whole slide images in diagnostic pathology. Am. J. Clin. Pathol. **130**, 259–264 (2008)
43. Varga, V.S., Ficsor, L., Kamaras, V., et al.: Automated multichannel fluorescent whole slide imaging and its application for cytometry. Cytometry A. **75**, 1020–1030 (2009)
44. Martina, J.D., Simmons, C., Jukic, D.M.: High-definition hematoxylin and eosin staining in a transition to digital pathology. J. Pathol. Inform. **2**, 45 (2011)
45. Webster, J.D., Michalowski, A.M., Dwyer, J.E., et al.: Investigation into diagnostic agreement using automated computer-assisted histopathology pattern recognition image analysis. J. Pathol. Inform. **3**, 18 (2012)
46. Bautista, P., Yagi, Y.: Digital simulation of staining in histopathology multispectral images: enhancement and linear transformation of spectral transmittance. J. Biomed. Opt. **17**, 05601310 (2012)
47. Tani, S.: Color standardization system implementing estimation method for absorption spectra of dye. Anal. Cell Pathol. **34**, 180 (2013)
48. Yagi, Y.: Color standardization and optimization in whole slide imaging. Diagn. Pathol. **6**, S15 (2011)
49. Keller, B., Chen, W., Gavrielides, M.A.: Quantitative assessment and classification of tissue-based biomarker expression with color content analysis. Arch. Pathol Lab. Med. **136**, 539–550 (2012)
50. Nederlof, M., Watanabe, S., Burnip, B., Taylor, D.L., Critchley-Thorne, R.: High-throughput profiling of tissue and tissue model microarrays: combined transmitted light and 3-color fluorescence digital pathology. J. Pathol. Inform. **2**, 50 (2011)
51. Hipp, J., Cheng, J., Pantanowitz, L., et al.: Image microarrays (IMA): digital pathology's missing tool. J. Pathol. Inform. **2**, 47 (2011)
52. Feldman, M.D.: Beyond morphology: whole slide imaging, computer-aided detection, and other techniques. Arch. Pathol. Lab. Med. **132**, 758–763 (2008)
53. Nanda, R.: Targeting the human epidermal growth factor receptor 2 (HER2) in the treatment of breast cancer: recent advances and future directions. Rev. Recent Clin. Trials **2**, 111–116 (2007)
54. Bautista, P.A., Hashimoto, N., Yagi, Y.: Color Standardization in whole slide imaging using a color calibration slide. J. Pathol. Inform. **5**, 4 (2014)
55. Hedvat, C.V.: Digital microscopy: past, present, and future. Arch. Pathol. Lab. Med. **134**, 1666–1670 (2010)
56. Dennis, T., Start, R.D., Cross, S.S.: The use of digital imaging, video conferencing, and telepathology in histopathology: a national survey. J. Clin. Pathol. **58**, 254–258 (2005)
57. Isaacs, M., Lennerz, J.K., Yates, S., et al.: Implementation of whole slide imaging in surgical pathology: a value added approach. J. Pathol. Inform. **2**, 39 (2011)
58. Tsuchihasi, Y.: Expanding application of digital pathology in Japan—from education, telepathology to autodiagnosis. Diagn. Pathol. **6**, S19 (2011)
59. Ho, J., Parwani, A., Jukic, D.M., et al.: Use of whole slide imaging in surgical pathology quality assurance: design and pilot validation studies. Hum. Pathol. **37**, 322–331 (2006)

References

60. Johnson, D.E.: NightHawk teleradiology services: a template for pathology? Arch. Pathol. Lab. Med. **132**, 745–747 (2008)
61. Cornish, T.C., Swapp, R.E., Kaplan, K.J.: Whole-slide imaging: routine pathologic diagnosis. Adv. Anat. Pathol. **19**, 152–159 (2012)
62. Evans, A., Sinard, J.H., Fatheree, L.A., Henricks, W.H., Carter, A.B., Contis, L., et al.: Validating whole slide imaging for diagnostic purposes in pathology: recommendations of the College of American Pathologists (CAP) pathology and laboratory quality centre. Anal. Cell. Pathol. **34**, 174 (2011)
63. Singh, R., Chubb, L., Pantanowitz, L., Parwani, A.: Standardization in digital pathology: supplement 145 of the DICOM standards. J. Pathol. Inform. **2**, 23 (2011)
64. Yagi, Y., Rojo, M.G., Kayser, K., et al.: The first congress of the international academy of digital pathology: digital pathology comes of age. Anal. Cell Pathol. Amst. **35**, 1–2 (2012)
65. McClintock, D.S., Lee, R.E., Gilbertson, J.R.: Using computerized workflow simulations to assess the feasibility of Whole Slide Imaging full adoption in a high volume histology laboratory. Anal. Cell Pathol. **34**, 182–184 (2013)
66. Amin, M., Sharma, G., Parwani, A.V., et al.: Integration of digital gross pathology images for enterprise-wide access. J. Pathol. Inform. **3**, 10 (2012)
67. Wang, F., Oh, T.W., Vergara-Niedermayr, C., Kurc, T., Saltz, J.: Managing and querying whole slide images. Proceedings of SPIE. pp. 83190J, (2012)
68. Wang, Y., Williamson, K.E., Kelly, P.J., James, J.A., Hamilton, P.W.: SurfaceSlide: a multitouch digital pathology platform. PLoS One **7**, e30783 (2012)
69. Hamilton, P.W., Wang, Y., McCullough, S.J.: Virtual microscopy and digital pathology in training and education. APMIS **120**, 305–315 (2012)
70. Schwartz, J.: Expanding the lab's reach with digital pathology. MLO Med. Lab. Obs. **43**, 41 (2011)

Chapter 2
Hardware and Software

Abstract Lest those interested in exploring the field not understand the nuts and bolts of the system, no book on digital technology is complete without some background on the available hardware and software. The field is changing rapidly, and specific examples may be already obsolete at the time this book goes to press. At the same time, we have found that certain principles have remained constant for a relatively long time now, and we believe that providing readers with some general technical background will help on the path to implementing successful digital pathology solutions.

Keywords Digital pathology · Slide scanner · Tile scanner · Line scanner · File format · Medical imaging · WSI · DP · MRXS · NDPI · SVS · BIF

This chapter talks about the technology that is used to arrive at digital pathology. As the pathologist is dependent upon his microscope, so is the digital pathologist dependent upon a digital camera or slide scanner for the creation of a single, high-magnification digital image of an entire microscopic slide or whole slide image (WSI).

This chapter is split into two parts. In Sect. 2.1, we elaborate on the various hardware components necessary to acquire virtual slides. In Sect. 2.2, we survey the various approaches to data storage and file format organization that different vendors have developed.

2.1 How Are Digital Pathology Images "Captured"?

Basically, WSI hardware consists of a robotic/automated microscope with specialized acquisition software. Some instruments are more specialized and purpose-specific in their design and construction than others. The simplest

---

An errartum to this chapter can be found under DOI 10.1007/978-3-319-08780-1_7

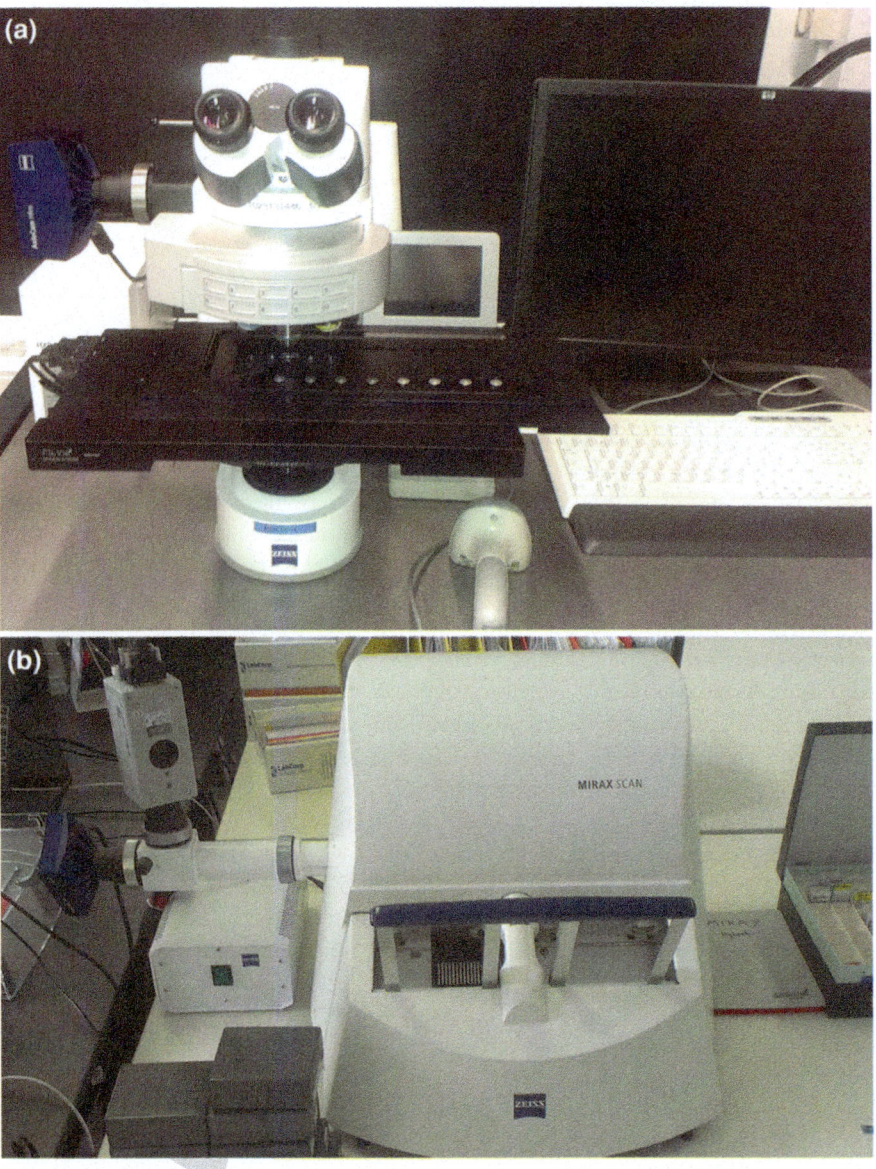

Fig. 2.1 a A Zeiss AxioVision setup with a mounted camera and robotic stage. **b** A 3DHistech high-volume slide scanner (courtesy of HistoGeneX)

setups consist of add-on cameras on top of conventional microscopes. This is a great start if all you want to do is capture regions of interest (ROIs) and share them with colleagues or embed them in your publications. However, they are not necessarily suited for whole slide imaging. In order to do WSI, as well as systematically digitize your entire workflow, you need at least a robotic staging table as well. The robot then cooperates with the software component to move the slide, capturing individual ROIs that then are stitched back together to generate a WSI. Special viewing software is usually provided so that it appears that a seamless image was obtained of the entire slide. As an alternative, there also are devices like microscopes with mounted cameras but automated stages. The advantage is that viewed ROIs can be stored even when you switch between different slides (Fig. 2.1).

Technology has by now become sufficiently specialized so that some companies only sell complete integrated systems (scanners). However, others sell individual components as well. Examples of the latter are Hamamatsu, which sells its own nanozoomer slide scanner as an integrated system, but also sells its components to TissueGnostics for their automated solutions.

2.2 How Do Slide Scanners Work?

Slide scanners are the highest level of abstraction for digital microscopy. They have both a hardware and software components. We distinguish five levels, from lowest to highest: slide handling, slide scanning, optics, detection, and, finally, acquisition software. These five levels are depicted in Fig. 2.2.

The first slide scanner was designed by James Bacus in 1994, during a period of rapid Internet expansion worldwide. The corresponding BLISS system, which is now recognized as having been the first virtual microscopy system ever developed, was designed to generate virtual microscope slides. Meanwhile, a WebSlide Server, Browser, and ActiveX Viewer were developed to allow for viewing virtual microscope slides over the Internet. Over the next several years, the Bacus group developed and patented the methods and apparati to perform automated assays of biological specimens, immunoploidy analysis, measurements of tissue thickness, and tests of neoplasm progression, as well as devices to allow for the remote control of microscopes, the creation of virtual microscopy slides, the magnification of specimen images, and the Internet, intranet, and local viewing of such slides [1–19]. Moreover, Bacus Laboratories not only created the first virtual slide system, they also created the first market for it. They did this by framing their system as an educational tool. Their plan was to ultimately replace standard microscopes with virtual microscopy in medical education. They achieved this by combining their virtual microscopy system with a collection of educational "slides," for which institutions could lease access licenses annually. Because of its successful business model, Bacus Laboratories was purchased by Olympus America Inc. in 2006.

In terms of features, the capacities of slide scanners today vary widely. For example, some can do bright-field images only, some can do fluorescence images only, and some can do both. The price of a model generally correlates with its slide-loading capacity, which can range from one to 400 slides per batch. Slides

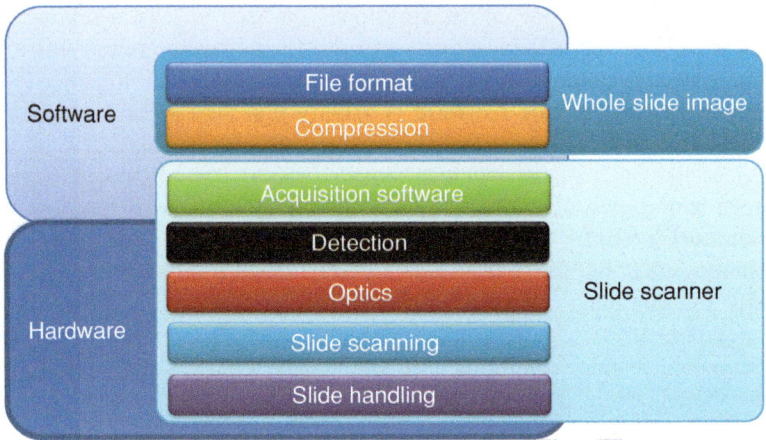

Fig. 2.2 Different layers of processing in digital pathology

can be handled as a single slide/stage, as standalone autoloaders ("hotels"), as slide trays, or as slide magazines. The type of slide can vary as well: While most scanners today still handle basic 1" × 3" slides only, others—like Aperio and Huron Technologies—also support 2" × 3" and even larger (whole mount) slides. The more variability that is allowed for physical slide media, the harder it is to batch process large numbers of slides.

Two approaches exist to scanning a slide: tile scanning (Bacus patents) [20] and line scanning (Aperio patents) [21]. In both cases, the resulting images (tiles or strips) are fitted together into a single large image (i.e., the WSI). With a tile scanner, the slide is scanned as a series of rectangular tiles. For each tile, the highest physical magnification desired is used (e.g., 40× or 20×). The tiles are then stacked into a WSI, like bricks forming a wall. This is done either concurrently with or after the scanning process, via the acquisition software. Conversely, with line scanning, after magnification, strips are combined side by side into a single image. Proponents of the latter approach claim that it generates fewer seams and, hence, fewer optical aberrations (Fig. 2.3).

One particular problem related to scanning is focusing. A pathologist looking through a microscope automatically adjusts the focus depending upon the area of the slide he or she is looking at, the thickness of the specimen, the type of glass slide used, etc. With a scanner, this process must be automated. With both tile and line scanners, it is possible to autofocus each field after moving the stage, but this can be very time-consuming, especially with tile scanners. A better approach is to focus on every nth field being scanned. This is both faster and simpler; but the placement of focus points lacks context, and it is still possible to waste time on larger areas that, by chance, do not require refocusing. A focus map is another solution. With this approach, focus points are distributed over the tissue forming a surface. Focus is only recalculated for intervening tissue. The number of selected

2.2 How Do Slide Scanners Work?

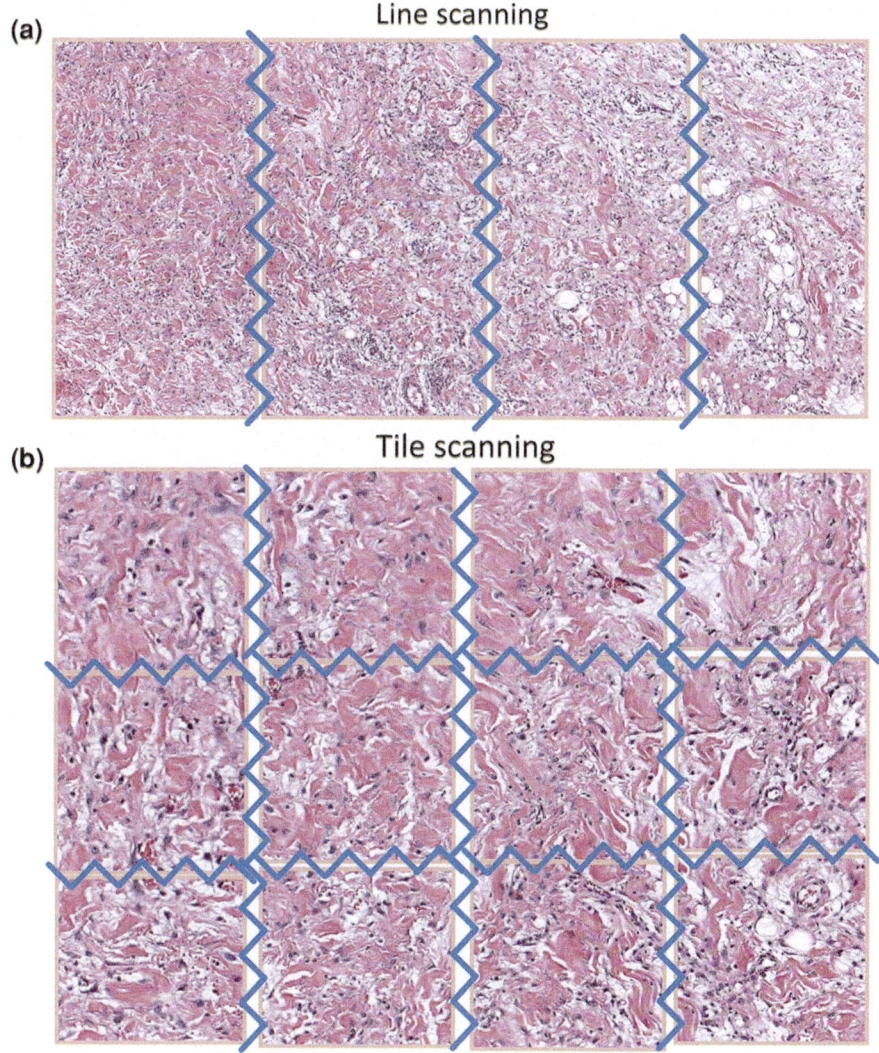

Fig. 2.3 a/b Line versus tile scanning: note the huge decrease in the number of seams with line scanning

focus points can be controlled via the scanner software. A trade-off is usually made between more focus points (less speed) and greater accuracy. The settings can be tissue dependent, and a technician can maintain a preset list of "profiles" that can be referred to, depending upon the type of specimen that needs to be scanned.

Z-stacking is becoming increasingly commonplace, but this poses its own unique challenges to file format organization (see later in this chapter). The new frontier is now spectral imaging.

2.3 Virtual Slide Formats

2.3.1 How Are WSI Data Organized?

After the acquisition software in the scanner obtains a digital image representation of a slide, it needs to store this information somewhere. This again can be seen as a two-step process, whereby first data compression takes place, and subsequently data are stored, usually in a vendor-specific file format.

Digital slide image formats typically consist of one or more files that contain high-resolution scanned areas as well as image information in the form of metadata. The resolution of such images varies, but usually ranges from ten to hundreds of thousands of pixels per dimension (width, height). Various techniques are currently employed to make it easier and quicker to process such images using computer software.

2.3.2 The Pyramidal Format

Scaled versions of the original image (called "zoom levels") are often created and stored in a single-"container" format. This is usually called a "pyramidal format," since every scaled-down image is smaller than its previous level, just like a pyramid gets smaller and smaller the higher up you go. By storing pre-computed scaled-down versions of the high-resolution image, a computer program can quickly render a smaller version of the image by reading pixel data from the zoom level closest to the scale currently being displayed (Fig. 2.4).

The pyramidal format increases display performance at the cost of storage efficiency. For this reason, many vendors try to minimize the actual scan area that is being stored. This is done by spotting the significant areas while scanning the slide and only storing these in high resolution. This leads to a digital slide image with many sparse high-resolution areas, which may follow the pyramidal format independently. For different tissue types, the tissue detection parameters (called "profiles" by some vendors) often must be fine-tuned.

2.3.3 Tiles

To further optimize random access and minimize disk read operations (input/output or I/O), digital slides split the image into smaller rectangular areas (tiles). Every zoom level is therefore a grid of tiles of the same size. When a computer program needs to display a small part of a high-resolution image, it is able to reduce the data being read by selecting only those tiles that intersect with the current viewport.

Slide scanning is performed in steps. The scanner's camera moves along the slide and takes pictures which are then stitched together by the scanner's software. Some

2.3 Virtual Slide Formats

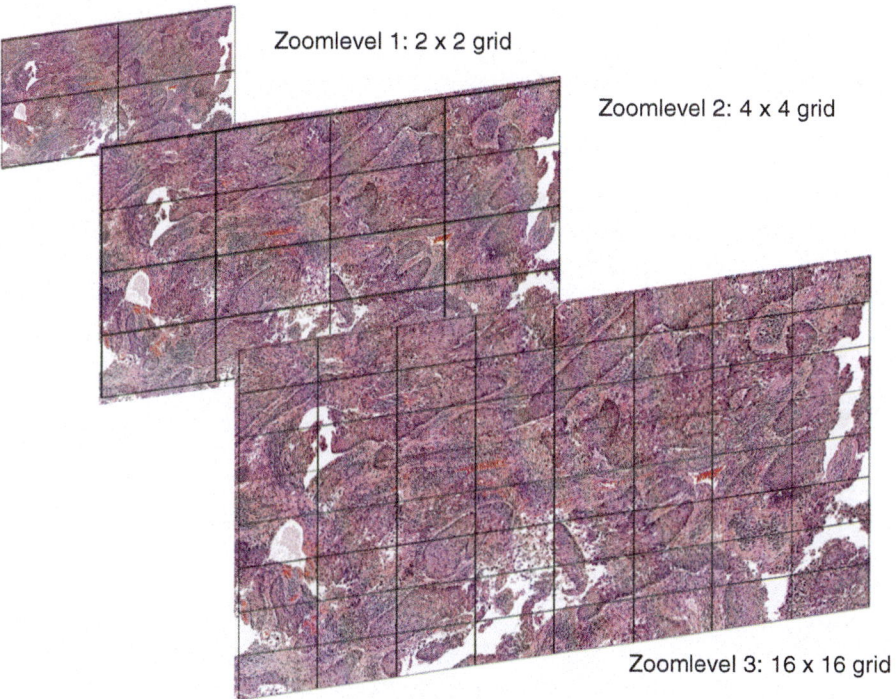

Fig. 2.4 A pyramidal stack represented symbolically on a sample whole slide image

vendors decide to store overlapping images of the slide and let the viewing software do the stitching. This is done because selecting stitching offsets that depend on the visible parts of the image every time may reduce stitching artifacts. This, in turn, would have otherwise been introduced if stitching had happened during scanning. In this case, stitching hints are stored as metadata along with the image.

Regardless of when the stitching process takes place (during scanning or while the image is viewed), images acquired by the scanner require adjustments. Overlapping regions might have differences in brightness and contrast, known as *shading*, due to the different positions of the camera each time a photograph is taken. Various techniques are employed to address this issue, such as blending and histogram equalization.

2.3.4 Color Spaces

The most common illumination techniques found in digital slides are bright-field and fluorescence. Bright-field microscopy images typically store pixels in the red, green, and blue (RGB) model (color space) or YC_BC_R (another family of color spaces) for JPEG images. Grayscale (points of equal RGB values; essentially a subspace of the RGB model) is especially used in the case of fluorescence microscopy slides to store the intensity of the reflected emission. This is then multiplied by a constant factor in order to be colorized for display purposes.

2.3.5 Compression Schemes

Digital pathology images employ various compression and image representation schemes, which may or may not lead to color information loss. Some of the compression schemes that are used are Raw, JPEG, JPEG2000, PNG, LZW, and DEFLATE.

2.4 Vendor-Specific File Format Implementations

The images that are generated by digital slide scanners are very different from the JPEG images typically obtained using your cell phone or digital camera. To start with, they are vastly larger and more complex. This is aptly demonstrated in Fig. 2.3, in which a typical high-resolution digital camera image is compared to a typical digital WSI. Note that the WSI has almost 1,500 times as many pixels (200,000 × 100,000 vs. 4,600 × 3,000) as the camera shot (Fig. 2.5).

There also are a large number of different WSI file formats, which are necessary because of the multiple applications for which these images are used, beyond simple viewing. For example, Zeiss format (czi and zvi) images (see further in this chapter) can encompass as many as six or seven dimensions, versus the 2-dimensional JPEG you generate with your home camera, to accommodate their use for microbiology, time lapse, fluorescence, and other applications. Below, we briefly describe just some of these various formats, highlighting their basic characteristics, as well as their advantages, disadvantages, and differences.

2.4.1 TIFF-Based Formats

2.4.1.1 TIFF

TIFF images are used by scanner vendors to store digital slides. The TIFF format natively supports storing images in grids of tiles and is generally well suited for random access. It allows for multiple images (directories) to be stored within a single file and for various compression schemes to be used. Since a slide's size may overcome the maximum 4 GB threshold, the BigTIFF format is also common. It essentially uses 64-bit pointers to store offsets within the file.

2.4 Vendor-Specific File Format Implementations

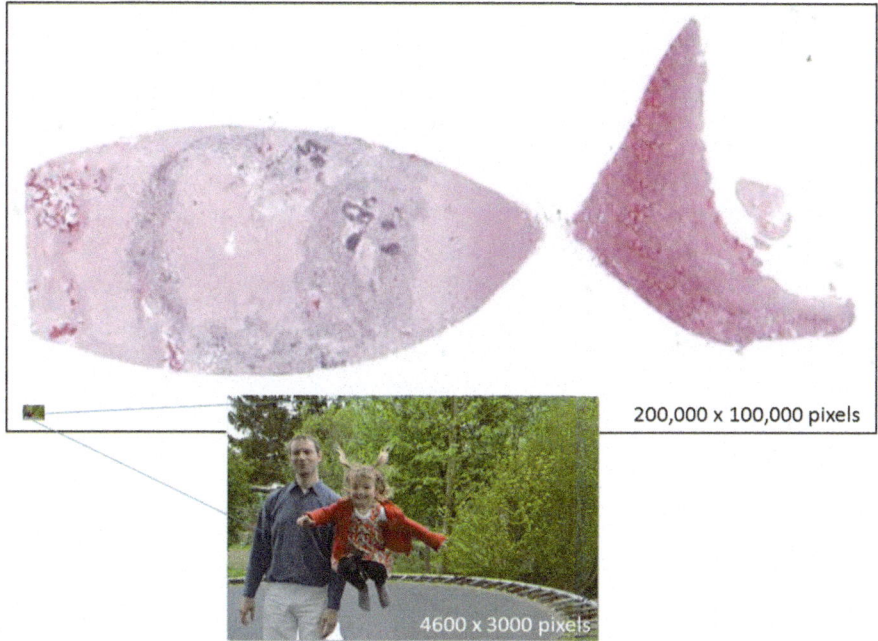

Fig. 2.5 Comparing a traditional high-resolution digital camera photograph (of coauthor YS and his bouncing daughter) against a typical digital whole slide image

A tiled TIFF directory specifies four important tags:

- Tile width (TIFF specifications tag number 322)
- Tile length (also known as height) (323)
- Tile offsets (324)
- Tile byte counts (325)

Typically, one TIFF directory is the high-resolution image, while several others may follow that are down-scaled versions of the original. One downside of the plain TIFF format is that there is no definitive way to specify which directory is for the high-resolution image and which are for the down-scaled images, because the specifications do not anticipate relationships between the directories. The display software attempts to overcome this by making assumptions; for example, the largest directory (in width or height) may be considered the original image and every other directory a smaller zoom level.

2.4.1.2 Open Microscopy Environment TIFF (Extensions .tif, .tiff)

The OME-TIFF format was created to maximize the respective strengths of OME-XML and TIFF. It takes advantage of the rich metadata defined in OME-XML, while retaining the pixels in multi-page TIFF format for compatibility with many more applications.

An OME-TIFF dataset has the following characteristics:

- Image planes are stored within one multi-page TIFF file, or across multiple TIFF files. Any image organization is feasible.
- A complete OME-XML metadata block describing the dataset is embedded within each TIFF file's header. Thus, even if some of the TIFF files in a dataset are misplaced, the metadata remain intact.
- The OME-XML metadata block may contain anything allowed in a standard OME-XML file.
- OME-TIFF uses the standard TIFF mechanism for storing one or more image planes in each of the constituent files, instead of encoding pixels as base 64 chunks within the XML. Since TIFF is an image format, it makes sense to only use OME-TIFF as opposed to OME-XML, when there is at least one image plane.

2.4.1.3 Leica SCN (Extension .scn)

Leica slides are stored in single-file BigTIFF format. The image description tag for the first TIFF directory contains an XML document that defines the structure of the slide. The slides are structured as a collection of images, each of which has multiple dimensions (pyramid levels). The collection has a size, and images have both a size and position. Each dimension has a size in pixels, an optional focal plane number, and a TIFF directory that contains the image data. Fluorescence images have different dimensions (and thus different TIFF directories) for each channel.

Bright-field slides have at least two images: a low-resolution macro-image and one or more main images corresponding to regions of the macro-image. The macro-image has a position of (0, 0) and a size that matches the size of the collection. Fluorescence slides can have two macro-images: one bright-field and one fluorescence.

2.4.1.4 Aperio SVS (Extension .svs)

Aperio slides are stored in single-file TIFF format. The first directory in an SVS file is always the full-resolution image. This image is always tiled, usually with a tile size of 240 × 240 pixels. The second image is always a thumbnail, typically with dimensions of about 1,024 × 768 pixels. Unlike the other slide images, the thumbnail image is always stored in strips, instead of tiles. Following the thumbnail, there may be one or more intermediate "pyramid" images. These are always compressed with the same type of compression as the baseline image and have a tiled organization of identical tile size.

Optionally at the end of an SVS file, there may be a slide label image, which is a low-resolution picture taken of the slide's label, and/or a macro-camera image, which is a low-resolution picture taken of the entire slide. The label and macro-images are always stored in strips.

2.4.1.5 Ventana BIF (Extension .bif)

Ventana slides are stored in single-file BigTIFF format. The first directory contains a label image, usually in tiled format. This is a thumbnail which includes the actual physical label for the glass slide. The directory specifies the XMP tag (700) and stores valid XML metadata about the slide. Next comes a thumbnail, and the high-resolution image follows.

BIF images contain overlapping tiles, and an appropriate algorithm is required to correctly render them. The directory containing the high-resolution images also specifies the XMP tag which contains tile stitching hints between neighboring tiles. The rendering algorithm calculates global coordinates for every tile, based on these hints. This may result in stitching artifacts in parts of the image. Subsequent image directories do not have such information, and tile positions are calculated via reduction to the base level.

2.4.1.6 Hamamatsu NDPI (Extension .ndpi)

Hamamatsu NDPI slides are stored in single-file TIFF format. Unlike other TIFF-based formats, NDPI does not use TIFF's tile format. Instead, every directory contains a single JPEG image, declared as stripped. These images are not necessarily valid. The JPEG specification does not allow images larger than $65,536 \times 65,536$ pixels. Therefore, when a directory exceeds these limits, NDPI sets the width and height of the image to zero. This means that at least some JPEG libraries are unable to read the image data. It is still possible to parse these with out-of-the-box solutions like a LIBJPEG. When doing so, the programmer has to invoke a callback mechanism to inform the JPEG decoder of the actual size whenever 0, 0 (a 'reset marker') is found in the stream.

Restart markers are placed inside the JPEG stream to achieve support for random-access reading. Each interval contains one tile, effectively implementing a tiled format within the JPEG image. The offsets of the markers are stored in a custom TIFF tag (65426), so that the whole stream does not need be parsed for them to be located.

2.4.2 Other Format Types

2.4.2.1 3DHISTECH Mirax (Extension .mrxs)

3DHISTECH Mirax slides are stored in a multi-file JPEG format with proprietary metadata and indexes. JPEG images are packed into a small number of data files, while the index file provides offsets into the data files for each required piece of data.

The camera on MIRAX scanners takes overlapping photographs and records the position of each one. Each photograph is then split into multiple JPEG images which do not overlap. Overlaps only occur between images that come from different photographs.

To generate level $n + 1$, each JPEG image from level n is down-sampled by two and then concatenated into a new JPEG image, with four old images per new JPEG image (2×2). This process is repeated for each level, irrespective of image overlaps. Therefore, at sufficiently high levels, a single image can contain one or more embedded overlaps of non-integral width.

2.4.2.2 Olympus VSI (Extensions .vsi, .ets)

The VSI file format is based on the well-known TIFF image file format. Besides the standard TIFF IFDs (image file directories) necessary to access the raster pixel data, the VSI format contains a chain of custom tags used to store additional information in the image files.

VSI files may contain multiple regions of the same physical slide, each scanned at a different level of resolution. High-resolution pixel data are not stored within the .vsi file, but in files with an .ets extension, stored in subdirectories defined within the VSI.

Extensible tile server (ETS) is a proprietary file format that is used to store multi-dimensional data organized in tiles. Usually, a single region of a slide is stored in tiled pyramidal fashion inside an ETS file.

2.4.2.3 Carl Zeiss CZI/ZISRAW (Extension .czi)

This format has been designed to be as close as possible to the open microscopy environment (OME) specification (http://www.openmicroscopy.org). The XML schema definition (XSD) was defined to exhibit maximum compatibility with the OME tiff and XML data formats, while maintaining the essential requirements to run Carl Zeiss ZEN software optimally.

The chosen architecture is a chain of "segments." Each segment is identified by a header with a defined identifier (SID). Segments are aligned on 32-byte boundaries. This improves the speed of the recovery process when rescanning the file, which can be useful in situations like when the system crashes. A single search step in case of a missing segment header can move to the next multiple of 32 bytes instead of advancing byte by byte.

2.4.2.4 Carl Zeiss ZVI (Extension .zvi)

The ZVI format is a standard OLE compound file containing a storage named "image" for the container image and commonly used information. The image data (pixel array) items are contained in substorages named "item(n)" where (n) is a value from 0 to Count − 1.

2.4.3 The Role of DICOM

As the proverbial 800-pound gorilla in the room, DICOM deserves its own paragraph. DICOM stands for *Digital Imaging and Communication in Medicine* and is a network maintained by the National Electronic Manufacturer's Association (NEMA) and supported by large-image management systems called *picture archive and communication systems* (PACS). Various PACS systems are used in hospitals and laboratories to manage images used for clinical and research purposes in medicine; this includes, among other functions, their storage and retrieval.

Since 2009, a new supplement has been added to the DICOM standard. This supplement is known as "Supp 145, Whole Slide Imaging in Pathology." The supplement was developed by Workgroup 26 and describes how an extension has been made to the DICOM standard to allow for the storage of very large images. The DICOM standard defines a family set for the image, called "instances" as per the DICOM vocabulary. All these instances follow an information object definition which is defined in PS 3.3; currently, version 2011 is the latest available. In all those IODs, DICOM instances have columns and rows defined as unsigned short values. What this means is that, in theory, all images must be 64K columns and rows. WSI frequently has images much larger than these pixel dimensions.

Rather than following what occurs during the TIFF to BigTIFF (64 bits extension) transition, the DICOM committee chose a different, very conservative approach, whereby the unsigned short value for the column and row does not change. Instead, new attributes are added to store the actual pixel dimension. In this scenario, a single WSI cannot be stored within a single "instance." Instead, a single WSI is inserted in fragments at a series level.

The proposed approach guarantees that all legacy software remains able to process any incoming WSI series, since the attributes in columns and rows are still defined as unsigned short.

One should notice, though, that this supplement pushes the DICOM standard to the edge, since uncompressed pixel data stored within a single DICOM instance are limited to a $2^{32} - 1$ byte (4 GB minus a byte, 0xFFFFFFFF being a reserved value). Therefore, the lower level of this pyramid is unlikely to be saved in uncompressed form, since its total size will likely exceed that limit considerably. In such a case, it is assumed that another transfer syntax will be used for those larger pyramid levels (e.g., JPEG). When using an encapsulated transfer syntax (e.g., JPEG type), there is no such limit, and all individual tiles can be stored within a single DICOM instance.

2.5 Bits, Bytes, and Wires

This book is not intended as guidelines on how you can build your own scanner or write your own WSI-viewer software. Nevertheless, no review of digital pathology can be complete without also addressing the hardware and software involved.

We have tried to introduce you to some of the intricacies of engineering that were required to develop slide scanners in the first place. Then, we moved on to the software side of things: How are WSI data stored? This is something that we all get exposed to, if only by transferring slides to a colleague via a USB memory key.

Slide scanners have not been around all that long. Two basic modes of operation exist for scanners, and virtually all scanners on the market today can be traced back to one or two sets of patents. Data captured by the slide scanner must be stored on the hard disk of the user's computer and organized so that it can be visualized optimally. File formats have been devised by different vendors to accomplish this. Because of the pixel size of the raw data (roughly 1,500 times more than the digital camera that you use on vacation) and the different features of the scanners (bright-field, fluorescence, confocal, etc.), various solutions have been thought of. However, these differences make it hard to move from one digital pathology platform to another, and one risks vendor lock-in because of this. Some initiatives for standardization have already been undertaken and are expected to become more center stage in the future.

References

1. Bacus, J.V., Bacus, J.W.: Method and apparatus for processing an image of a tissue sample microarray. US Patent 6,466,690 (2000)
2. Bacus, J.V., Bacus, J.W.: Method and apparatus for acquiring and reconstructing magnified specimen images from a computer-controlled microscope. US Patent 6,101,265 (2000)
3. Bacus, J.V., Bacus, J.W.: Method and apparatus for acquiring and reconstructing magnified specimen images from a computer-controlled microscope. US Patent 6,226,392 (2001)
4. Bacus, J.V., Bacus, J.W.: Method and apparatus for creating a virtual microscope slide. US Patent 6,272,235 (2001)
5. Bacus, J.V., Bacus, J.W.: Method and apparatus for acquiring and reconstructing magnified specimen images from a computer-controlled microscope. US Patent 6,404,906 (2002)
6. Bacus, J.V., Bacus, J.W.: Apparatus for remote control of a microscope. US Patent 6,674,884 (2004)
7. Bacus, J.V., Bacus, J.W.: Method and apparatus for creating a virtual microscope slide. US Patent 6,775,402 (2004)
8. Bacus, J.V., Bacus, J.W.: Apparatus for remote control of a microscope. US Patent 7,110,586 (2006)
9. Bacus, J.V., Bacus, J.W.: Method and apparatus for creating a virtual microscope slide. US Patent 7,146,372 (2006)
10. Bacus, J.V., Bacus, J.W.: Method and apparatus for internet, intranet, and local viewing of virtual microscope slides. US Patent 7,149,332 (2006)
11. Bacus, J.W., Bacus, J.V.: Method and apparatus for automated assay of biological specimens. US Patent 5,473,706 (1995)
12. Bacus, J.W.: Method and apparatus for automated analysis of biological specimens. US Patent 5,526,258 (1996)
13. Bacus, J.W., Marder, J.M.: Method and apparatus for immunoploidy analysis. US Patent 5,541,064 (1996)
14. Bacus, J.W., Bacus, J.V.: Method and apparatus for measuring tissue section thickness. US Patent 5,546,323 (1996)

References

15. Bacus, J.W., Oud, P.S.: Apparatus and method for analysis of biological specimens. US Patent 5,485,527 (1996)
16. Bacus, J.W., Bacus, J.V.: Method and apparatus for testing a progression of neoplasia including cancer chemoprevention testing. US Patent 6,031,930 (2000)
17. Bacus, J.W., Bacus, J.V.: Method and apparatus for internet, intranet, and local viewing of virtual microscope slides. US Patent 6,396,941 (2002)
18. Bacus, J.W., Bacus, J.V.: Method and apparatus for creating a virtual microscope slide. US Patent 6,522,774 (2003)
19. Bacus, J.W., Bacus, J.V.: Method and apparatus for internet, intranet, and local viewing of virtual microscope slides. US Patent 6,674,881 (2004)
20. James W.: Bacus patents. JamesBacus.com. (2014). Ref type: Electronic Citation
21. Aperio Technologies Inc., Patent Applications. Patentdocs. (2014). Ref type: Electronic Citation

Chapter 3
Applications

Abstract Despite the diverse appearances and usage scenarios, digital pathology applications can nevertheless be categorized into a number of distinct topics and fields. In this chapter, we start with the most obvious of these applications and move toward the least obvious. We limit ourselves to explaining the field of applications here. In practice, applied digital pathology most likely involves a combination of applications, as can be seen in Chap. 5, where we highlight certain specific use cases.

Keywords Digital pathology · Pathology applications · Primary diagnosis · Second opinion · Pathology education · Quality assurance · Tumor board · Biobank · DP

3.1 Education

Whole slide imaging is increasingly being used for a number of applications. In education, for instance, WSI has been successfully adopted for graduate education in medical, dentistry, and veterinary schools, for the training of pathology residents, as an educational tool in cytotechnology, for virtual tracking and tutoring, at tumor boards, and on examinations [1].

Education may very well be the area in which the application of digital pathology is easiest, with the lowest risk, yet at the same time offering a high payoff. Every year, thousands of students go through a variety of histology and pathology courses. Viewing reference slides is expected to prepare them for their future careers. While high-quality slide sets exist, they are expensive and are typically not available to everyone. Oftentimes, a waterfall system is installed, whereby the best slides are used by medical school students, and more worn slides are used by nursing school students. Those slides that are the most worn—typically consisting of incomplete collections—end up in bachelors-level anatomy and physiology courses.

The reasons for this are practical, as well as economic: It takes a lot of time and effort to develop high-quality reference slides. Purchasing them from a third party is an alternative to save time, but obviously has a financial cost associated with it. Depending on the histological condition/disease that one wants (or needs) to capture, it may be more difficult (and more costly) to obtain the right slides, as well. With purchased slides, one does not usually get a sufficient number of identical slides (sliced at same level or even the same tissue sample) for a large class. Such variability makes teaching difficult. "Look for…" or "it resembles…" do not apply to all students' slides. With WSI, all students will have the same slide.

Once the slides are available, they are only available to a limited number of lecturers or students at a given time. During histology laboratory sessions, students typically must pass slides from one station to the next. Even with a multi-head microscope, there is limited viewing time (and multi-heads require frequent calibration, as well). In addition, coverslips become smudged, and occasionally slides break or are dropped due to improper (or careless) handling.

Compare this with a collection of digital slides. The slides are always available at any time to as many concurrent users as needed (albeit, limited by computer network and server constraints). Since slides no longer need to be physically handled, they cannot break or be dropped or misplaced. Furthermore, they do not fade or degrade over time. Assuming that quality assurance (QA) occurs before digital replicas are included in the reference collection, the colors will be as true and vibrant 10 years from now as they were on the 1 day the slides were stained. On the other hand, image color and quality vary, depending on the settings and quality of the student's computer/laptop. In a survey of screens during an actual digital pathology classroom session, one cannot deny that different students will observe very different presentations.

The construction of a collection for teaching purposes or as a reference set becomes easier as well, once the digital route is chosen. The preparation of physical glass slides for preservation purposes requires more attention to detail than is prescribed in daily pathology laboratory practices. This brings up an interesting dilemma (which also explains the high cost of purchasing these off the shelf): A prepared slide needs to be examined before inclusion. Clearly, not all slides will "make the cut," which means that a lot of effort and time is lost in preparing unfit slides. At the same time, interesting cases may turn up occasionally that are unfortunately unfit for inclusion, because the wrong preparation protocol was used. Contrast and compare this to going digital, with which any slide of interest that passes through a pathology or research laboratory can now be flagged, scanned, and included in any collection. Finally, a large number of digital WSI collections can also be accessed at other institutions.

Two great examples of WSI use in action within a medical education context are detailed in Chap. 5, the first at the New York College of Podiatric Medicine (NYCPM), and the second at the Italian Hospital in Cairo.

3.2 Remote Consultations and Second Opinions

Telepathology is probably the oldest form of digital pathology, especially since the practice need not necessarily incorporate digital pathology. Different types of telepathology exist: The content can be static or dynamic (either with or without robotic control), and combinations of static (reference) content and dynamic content exist as well. Whole (virtual) slide imaging is the most recent addition to the portfolio. WSI is nevertheless not a "capture it all" replacement for what existed previously: While virtual slides can be saved and edited, a mounted camera, converted into a video stream, can be sent to any remote site in a similar fashion that cable television signals are distributed. As such, the requirements for digital pathology are probably more demanding than for telepathology.

The benefits of telepathology systems are numerous and include enhancing medical services, allowing for increased specialization, saving money and time, enhancing both teaching and learning, and facilitating the exchange of knowledge. In terms of costs, the average cost of sending physical slides to only one American or European center (approximately US$100) plus the average fee for the consultation (approximately US$150) imply that the total costs for consulting on our specialized complex cases for this one center was US$12.500 annually. As usually two or three centers are consulted for each case to gather more opinions, this figure should be multiplied two to three times, up to US$37.500 annually. Compare this to the cost, once a digital system is set up, of a few simple mouse clicks to send images digitally.

Transmitted images may be used for multiple purposes, including aiding in establishing primary diagnoses, collecting second opinions, facilitating QA, testing personnel and system proficiency. Offsite learning is another application, which includes learning at "extreme" distances. The latter applies particularly to developing countries, which may lack sufficient resources or personnel to establish and maintain their own high-quality pathology services.

Preparation for telepathology requires several steps. Costs need to be evaluated, and funds to cover them need to be identified. Depending on which location one is in, the best available and qualified instruments need to be identified. This is not always straightforward, as telepathology is often deployed in remote and/or underdeveloped regions of the world. Practicality is therefore an important factor to consider, and it may be desirable to select somewhat less advanced equipment that is easier to operate or more durable. Furthermore, a consensus must be reached on the software that will be used, and the availability of connections for sending and receiving (live) data-feeds must be verified. A problem that is unique to digital pathology is its bandwidth requirements. At the 2013 20th International DICOM conference in Bangalore, India, several practitioners of rural medicine were pleading for applications that could also run over limited bandwidth (such as dial-up or ISDN). This is still a challenge for digital pathology, as color image streams are more difficult to compress. This may actually limit the application of digital pathology initially.

Once in place, however, service can be provided to any pathology department at any university, any research center, and any pathologist. Digital pathology allows for the creation of a countrywide and international network for clinical and teaching purposes, as well as for research. Asynchronous viewing also becomes possible, in that two or more pathologists can view and comment on the same slide on their own time, rather than having to coordinate so that the slides are viewed together.

3.3 Tumor Boards and Pathology Reviews

A tumor board can be defined as a group of physicians ± other healthcare providers with different specialties meeting to discuss specific cancer patients to determine the best course of management. Typically, this includes medical, surgical, and radiation oncologists [2], though other specialists may become involved as well; for example, a general internist may be included to provide input on comorbid diseases or a psychologist or social worker to address personal and interpersonal issues. Such boards have been in use for decades, the first description of one having been published as early as 1952 [3]. However, recently, there has been a push not only to increase their use, but to systematize them to enhance patient outcomes [2–5]. The rationale behind such boards is obvious: If two heads are better than one, why not have three or more extremely experienced and well-educated heads come together with the common goal of optimizing patient management? In recent years, such an approach is starting to fit particularly well with the emerging concept of "individualized" patient care, especially in light of so many cancer biomarkers and genomics-based therapies [6–9]. This inevitably increases the role of histopathology in treatment-related decisions.

In the past, tumor boards had little choice but to meet in person, usually at a hospital where most members, if not all, had their practices. But with teleconferencing and communication networks such as Skype now viable options, this is no longer as necessary. Such technology, combined with digital pathology, allows specialists miles and sometimes even countries apart to "meet" while having the slides in question immediately visible and interpretable (e.g., with pathologist annotations) right before them on their computer screens [5]. Even when boards do meet in person, it is helpful to have digital slides ± pathologist annotations available for review. Nonetheless, the ability to have virtual tumor boards creates countless opportunities for collaborations between departments, hospitals, and even countries [2].

Another tumor board-like application relates to research, especially in the context of multicenter clinical trials or cohort studies, which often are required when studying rare forms of cancer and/or rare outcomes (e.g., an uncommon but serious side effect of a drug or other treatment). Since such studies often involve centers some distance apart, sometimes in separate countries, having collaborators meet in person to collectively decide upon patient eligibility often is infeasible. And yet, the more assured everyone is that every subject entered into the study is truly appropriate for entry, the more confident the investigators themselves will

3.3 Tumor Boards and Pathology Reviews

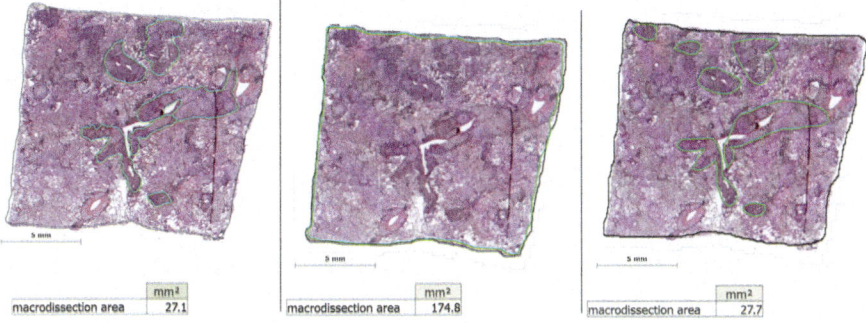

Fig. 3.1 Observations on the same tissue sample from three different pathologists

be—as well as grant application reviewers, journal reviewers and, ultimately, readers—that the ultimate results are generalizable to real-life practice. Digital pathology allows for collaborators from multiple centers to agree upon a histological diagnosis by all seeing, or having all their departments of pathology review, relevant slides. This helps them to reach a consensus regarding a given patient's eligibility for the study and, in studies in which the treatment arms entail some degree of flexibility, the most appropriate course of action.

WSI also is expected to play an important role in central pathology reviews, both in clinical trial settings and in second-opinion cases. This is likely to result in a substantial reduction in the overall turnaround time required for slide reviews at central locations [10].

Interesting extensions lie in the recruitment of new pathologists and in the evaluation of practicing pathologists. It can also offer a novel way of choosing pathology service providers. Figure 3.1 shows annotated lung tissue. Three pathologists were asked to select appropriate regions for macro-dissection, assuming subsequent downstream DNA extraction for mutation analysis. Clearly, the three pathologists came to different conclusions. This exercise can have far-reaching implications for the patient: Indicating the wrong area for mutation analysis can lead to misdiagnosis and the patient receiving incorrect therapy.

3.4 Biobanking and Collection Hosting

Translational biomedical research is based on large collections of high-quality samples combined with large sets of well-documented, up-to-date epidemiological, clinical, and/or molecular data from large numbers of patients and controls. Such collections are of the utmost importance in both investigator-driven and company-driven clinical trials. Biobanks are therefore considered essential for the advancement of research and development in the life sciences [11–17]. The term "biobank" is generally defined as an organized collection of human biological material and associated information stored for research purposes. As the term infers, collections of plants, animals, microbes, and other non-human materials could also be labeled biobanks. However, the term is generally reserved for collections of human specimens. Specimen types include blood (in all its forms; e.g., serum, plasma, isolated PBMCs), urine, saliva, skin cells, organ tissue, and other materials taken from the body. Specialized biobanks exist, such as the Network for Pancreatic Organ Donors with Diabetes (nPOD) biobank that houses pancreatic tissues (http://www.jdrfnpod.org) and biobanks that focus on heart valves. The primary task of the biobank is to maintain specimens in good condition for future analysis. For this purpose, biobanks usually have cryogenic storage facilities for the samples, ranging in size from individual refrigerators to warehouses, maintained by institutions such as hospitals, universities, and other non-profit organizations [11–21], but also by pharmaceutical companies (e.g., Astra Zeneca Global Biobank). Disease-oriented biobanks, usually located at a university-based hospital, often have formalin-fixed paraffin-embedded (FFPE) tissue available, next to fresh frozen tissue. Although many collections of human biological materials are present in European countries, these collections often suffer from (geographical) fragmentation, undefined access rules, lack of uniform quality standards, and the absence of any uniform legal and/or ethical framework, thereby hampering international collaboration.

Increasingly, the focus of cancer therapy is shifting toward personalized medicine. For optimal application of targeted molecular drugs, an improved understanding of the underlying molecular mechanisms may help to identify biomarkers that can be used clinically to predict response and establish new treatment options to overcome resistance. For this kind of research, FFPE tissue is the specimen most widely available. Moreover, in contrast with prospective studies, long-term clinical follow-up is an implied characteristic of a biobank. However, the use of high-quality, fresh-frozen biospecimens with appropriate clinical annotation would be preferable. Collections of human biological materials together with associated clinical data are key resources when investigating genetic and environmental factors underlying (multi-factorial) disease, with the aim of improving diagnosis and treatment and ultimately preventing or mitigating disease.

To provide a forum to address the integration of scientific, technical, legal, and ethical issues relevant to repositories of biological and environmental specimens, the International Society of Biological and Environmental Repositories (ISBER, http://www.isber.org) and its chapter covering the region encompassing Europe, the Middle-East, and Africa (ESBB, http://www.esbb.org) were established. These societies aim to create opportunities for sharing ideas and innovations in biobanking, as well as the harmonization of approaches to evolving challenges for biological and environmental repositories. Educational resources and meetings focus on technical issues such as QA and control, regulation, human subject privacy, and confidentiality issues and provide information about sources of equipment and expertise.

However, despite the development of strict protocols for the inclusion of material into biorepositories, specimens may still prove to be of little value for downstream testing. In one large study investigating 1,138 samples from the University of Indiana tissue bank, only 59 % were found to be at least 65 % tumor versus non-neoplastic tissue. Meanwhile, 23 % had a tumor volume that accounted for less than 65 % of the gross specimen, 17 % was entirely negative for tumor, and 1 % was completely necrotic. These findings underscore the importance of instituting adequate measures for histological sample quality control before the release of banked samples for downstream testing [22]. In fact, the availability of an online database of whole slide images for all specimens in a biobank would make it possible for researchers to preselect specimens based on tissue composition.

Finally, a fully digital workflow within pathology departments is within reach [23]. Since whole slide imaging is increasingly used for applications such as education and pathology reviews, it is likely that more laboratories will have access to digital pathology systems which will make whole slide image repositories as add-ons of existing biorepositories more feasible and, in the long term, even mandatory. A whole slide image database accompanying biorepositories should therefore be feasible. This can be taken even one step further by combining WSIs with digital pathology. Image analysis tools can be used to derive objective quantification measures from digital slides. Pattern recognition and visual search tools can be used to classify specimen imagery and identify medically significant regions of digital slides. Incorporating digital pathology into biobank QA procedures, using automated pattern recognition morphometric image analysis to quantify tissue features in digital WSI of tissue sections, can minimize the variability and subjectivity associated with routine pathologic evaluations in biorepositories. Whole slide images and pathologist-reviewed morphometric analyses can be provided to researchers to guide specimen selection [24]. As a specific example, unique spatial–spectral algorithms were developed for applying automated pattern recognition morphometric image analysis to quantify histological tumor and non-tumor tissue areas in biospecimen tissue sections. Measurements were acquired successfully for 75/75 (100 %) lymphomas, 76/77 (98.7 %) osteosarcomas, and 60/70 (85.7 %) melanomas. The percentage of tissue area occupied by tumor varied among patients and tumor types and was distributed around medians of 94 % for lymphomas, 84 % for melanomas, and 39 % for osteosarcomas. Within-patient comparisons from a subset, including multiple individual patient specimens, revealed $\leq$12 % median coefficient of variation (CV) for lymphomas and melanomas. However, due to phenotypic heterogeneity, the median CV for osteosarcomas was much higher. These data suggest that quantitative image analysis automation can minimize variability associated with routine biorepository pathologic evaluations and enhance biomarker discovery by helping to guide the selection of study-appropriate specimens [25]. An online histopathology system will be an important tool in the valorization of any biobank sample collection. An excellent example is the previously mentioned tissue repository installed by the nPOD-JDRF consortium (www.jdrfnpod.org), an initiative of the Juvenile Diabetes Research Foundation International, a large US patient organization. nPOD biobank houses pancreatic tissues from several hundred organ donors, including patients with diabetes [26]. It has proven to be a highly efficient concept that has attracted researchers and industry from all over the world. The online repository not only provides detailed patient data, including donor demographics and laboratory assays, it also permits digital microscopy access to scanned slides, allowing potential customers to choose and inspect tissue and patient characteristics before ordering tissue sections via their online system [27].

3.5 Primary Diagnosis

Primary diagnosis has been described by some as the Holy Grail of digital pathology. However, like the mythical artifact, it has been difficult to achieve.

3.5.1 In the USA: The Role of the FDA

Under the Food, Drug, and Cosmetic Act, the US Food and Drug Administration (FDA) recognizes three classes of medical device, based upon the level of control necessary to ensure their safety and effectiveness [28]. Classification procedures are described in the Code of Federal Regulations, Title 21, part 860 (usually known as 21 CFR 860) [29]. Class I devices are those that the FDA deems safe for use with minimal regulatory control. They generally are not intended to help support or sustain life or to be substantially important in preventing impairment to human health and are believed not to place patients at any unreasonable risk of illness or injury. Examples of Class I devices include elastic bandages, examination gloves, and handheld surgical instruments. Class III devices, meanwhile, are those devices the FDA deems most in need of regulatory control. Unlike Class I devices, they can help support or sustain life or be substantially important in preventing impairment to human health and could place patients at an unreasonable risk of illness or injury. Examples include implantable pacemakers, pulse generators, and diagnostic HIV tests.

Laboratories in the USA are currently prevented from using digital pathology for primary diagnosis, because the FDA has ruled that digital pathology is a Class III medical device. This is in contrast with traditional microscopes, which are considered a Class I medical device.

Some in the community are rather upset with this decision, because it arguably impedes the progress that can be made integrating digital pathology into daily practice. At the same time, however, the FDA had very good reasons to rule the way it did.

The reason that WSI is deemed to require a more comprehensive approach is that a traditional microscope is one component in a diagnostic system that only involves a light source and imaging optics. In contrast, WSI involves a slide scanner before the traditional microscope, followed by digital image capturing techniques, followed by the use of image processing software. These image acquisition, processing, and display capabilities are new technology with respect to the clinical assessment of tissue sections. Therefore, WSI systems cannot be considered Class I exempt.

The FDA is also not blind to reality. It recognizes that the technological advances associated with WSI make its use a reality and makes no attempt to regulate or comment upon any of the other applications mentioned earlier in this chapter.

At the end of the day it means that, before being embedded into daily clinical practice, since WSI systems are not Class I exempt, they are subject to premarket requirements. Current in vitro diagnostic tests (IVDs) that utilize digital imaging for limited applications are not applicable to the WSI paradigm.

It is hoped that parallels can be drawn with other areas of medicine that already have gone through digitization. Digital mammography may provide useful lessons, but does not address all of the concerns that exist for WSI. One problem is that, in order to speed up performance and reduce scan time, scanners do a pre-scan of a sample and auto-detect the presence of tissue. They then only scan the areas that they assume have tissue on them. Lightly stained areas can be missed in this way, and to date, there is no good way, besides manual inspection, to determine whether a scanner has indeed scanned all the tissue within a section under investigation. One of the main concerns of the FDA is that this process can result in the omission of diagnostically relevant tissue and thereby impact patient management.

Such issues should not prohibit parties from starting to explore digital pathology. Though the FDA has a say in the application of technology to US patients, a US laboratory can still apply digital pathology techniques for primary diagnosis in patients located outside the USA. We have observed many examples of this, both in profit and non-profit scenarios. It is interesting to note that, in an interesting twist on the outsourcing paradigm, a laboratory in the USA can now serve very well as a nighthawk service for developing countries, whereas traditionally this has occurred in the other direction.

3.5.2 Throughout the Rest of the World

At conferences, it is clear that digital pathology is starting to be used for primary diagnosis elsewhere. In some cases, practitioners want to adopt its use before a regulatory framework is in place, hoping to establish best practices from which regulations can follow, rather than the other way around.

The University Health Network (UHN) in Toronto, Canada, is at the forefront of this. Over the course of a decade, they have fully adopted the practice of digital pathology, one digital pathology niche at a time [30, 31]. Each implementation step was brought on by a specific need; but no particular application involved a huge volume of slides/cases at any given time. Therefore, it was possible to build up expertise and learn necessary lessons along the way, before eventually scaling up to handle larger volumes.

In 2004, an initial program was started for frozen section telepathology. Learning from its successes and failures, the program was expanded to transplant biopsy telepathology in 2007. In 2012, a collaboration was set up with the Kuwait Cancer Control Center. Also by 2012, slides were being routinely scanned at 20X, and 300–400 slides were being sent to UNH on a daily basis. By 2013, the center received 600–800 slides per day for primary diagnosis.

Over the period between November 2012 and August 2013, almost 10,000 slides were evaluated digitally, of which only about 3 % were deferred to glass review. Reasons for the latter varied and included pathologists still getting accustomed to working digitally, IT performance issues, the difficulty of the particular cases, and sub-optimal image quality or poor focus of the scanned area under investigation [30].

3.6 Birds of a Feather

While digital pathology is definitely a niche in the medical imaging universe, its applications can be wide and diverse. In this chapter, we have categorized the most important domains in which digital pathology plays a role. In practice, we find that most installations combine two or more of these. This is logical outflow from the fact that once the hardware is in place, it is usually versatile enough to facilitate various scenarios. One example is a university that not only uses digital pathology for second opinions from specialists, but also for teaching histology in its medical school, In addition, the pathology department might run an outreach program with another country. There is one big use case for digital pathology that we have not yet discussed, but that we feel is important enough to warrant its own chapter.

References

1. Huisman, A.: Digital pathology for education. Stud. Health Technol. Inform. **179**, 68–71 (2012)
2. El Saghir, N.S., Keating, N.L., Carlson, R.W., Khoury, K.E., Fallowfield, L.: Tumor boards: optimizing the structure and improving efficiency of multidisciplinary management of patients with cancer worldwide. Am. Soc. Clin. Oncol. Educ. Book **34**, e461–e466 (2014)
3. Bell, D.F. Jr.: The tumor board and tumor clinic at the children's hospital, Washington, D.C. Clin. Proc. Child. Hosp. Dist. Columbia **8**, 21–23 (1952)
4. Shah, S., Arora, S., Atkin, G., et al.: Decision-making in colorectal cancer tumor board meetings: results of a prospective observational assessment. Surg. Endosc. 1–6 (2014) [Epub ahead of print]
5. Marshall, C.L., Petersen, N.J., Naik, A.D., et al.: Implementation of a regional virtual tumor board: a prospective study evaluating feasibility and provider acceptance. Telemed. J. E Health. (2014) [Epub ahead of print]
6. Marquardt, J.U., Thorgeirsson, S.S.: Next-generation genomic profiling of hepatocellular adenomas: a new era of individualized patient care. Cancer Cell **25**, 409–411 (2014)
7. Harbour, J.W., Chen, R.: The decisionDx-UM gene expression profile test provides risk stratification and individualized patient care in Uveal Melanoma. PLoS Curr. (2013) Apr 9; 5. pii:ecurrents.eogt.af8ba80fc776c8f1ce8f5dc485d4a618. doi:10.1371/currents.eogt.af8ba80fc776c8f1ce8f5dc485d4a618

8. Vuong, D., Simpson, P.T., Green, B., Cummings, M.C., Lakhani, S.R.: Molecular classification of breast cancer. Virchows Arch. (2014) [Epub ahead of print]
9. Roundtable on Translating Genomic-Based Research for Health, Board on Health Sciences Policy, and Institute of Medicine. Refining processes for the co-development of genome-based therapeutics and companion diagnostic tests: Workshop summary. National Academies Press (US), Washington (DC). The National Academies Collection: Reports funded by National Institutes of Health (2014)
10. Slodowska, J., Garcia-Rojo, M.: Digital pathology in personalized cancer therapy. Stud. Health Technol. Inform. **179**, 143–154 (2012)
11. Hawkins, A.K.: Biobanks: importance, implications and opportunities for genetic counselors. J. Genet. Couns. **19**, 423–429 (2010)
12. Brand, A.M., Probst-Hensch, N.M.: Biobanking for epidemiological research and public health. Pathobiology **74**, 227–238 (2007)
13. Erichsen, R., Lash, T.L., Hamilton-Dutoit, S.J., et al.: Existing data sources for clinical epidemiology: the Danish National Pathology Registry and Data Bank. Clin. Epidemiol. **2**, 51–56 (2010)
14. Forsti, A., Hemmenki, K.: Breast cancer genomics based on biobanks. Methods Mol Biol. **675**, 375–385 (2011)
15. Hewitt, R., Hainaut, P.: Biobanking in a fast moving world: an international perspective. J. Natl. Cancer Inst. Monogr. **2011**, 50–51 (2011)
16. Marodin, G., Salgueiro, J.B., Motta Mda, L., Santos, L.M.: Brazilian guidelines for biorepositories and biobanks of human biological material. Rev. Assoc. Med. Bras. **59**, 72–77 (2013) [Article in English, Portuguese]
17. Caenazzo, L., Tozzo, P., Pegoraro, R.: Biobanking research on oncological residual material: a framework between the rights of the individual and the interest of society. BMC Med. Ethics **14**, 17 (2013)
18. Auray-Blais, C., Patenaude, J.: A biobank management model applicable to biomedical research. BMC Med. Ethics **7**, E4 (2006)
19. Mitchell, R.: National biobanks: clinical labor, risk production, and the creation of biovalue. Sci. Technol. Human Values **35**, 330–355 (2010)
20. Anderlik, M.: Commercial biobanks and genetic research: ethical and legal issues. Am. J. Pharmacogenomics, **3**, 203–215 (2003)
21. Kang, B., Park, J., Cho, S., et al.: Current status, challenges, policies, and bioethics of biobanks. Genomics Inform. **11**, 211–217 (2013)
22. Garcia Rojo, M.: State of the art and trends for digital pathology. Stud. Health Technol. Inform. **179**, 15–28 (2012)
23. Song, Y., Treanor, D., Bulpitt, A.J., Magee, D.R.: 3D reconstruction of multiple stained histology images. J. Pathol. Inform. **4**, S7 (2013)
24. Wells, C.A., Sowter, C.: Telepathology: a diagnostic tool for the millennium? J. Pathol. **191**, 1–7 (2000)
25. Coleman, R.: Can histology and pathology be taught without microscopes? The advantages and disadvantages of virtual histology. Acta Histochem. **111**, 1–4 (2009)
26. nPOD: Developing a tissue Biobank for T1D. Juvenile Diabetes Research Foundation (JDRF) (2014)
27. Campbell-Thompson, M., Wasserfall, C., Kaddis, J., et al.: Network for pancreatic organ donors with diabetes (nPOD): developing a tissue biobank for type 1 diabetes. Diabetes Metab. Res. Rev. **28**, 608–617 (2012)
28. Medical Devices: U.S. Food and Drug Administration (2014)
29. CFR—Code of Federal Regulations Title 21: U.S. Food and Drug Administration (2014)
30. Evans, A.J.: Whole slide imaging for primary diagnosis: a comprehensive concordance study in genitourinary pathology [slide presentation] (2014)
31. Tetu, B., Evans, A.: Canadian licensure for the use of digital pathology for routine diagnoses: one more step toward a new era of pathology practice without borders. Arch. Pathol. Lab. Med. **138**, 302–304 (2014)

Chapter 4
Image Analysis

Abstract In the field of digital pathology, image analysis refers to the computer-aided diagnostic assessment of whole slide images (WSIs). While image analysis is clearly another application of WSI, we feel that the subject has become vast enough to warrant its own chapter. The potential of digital pathology has taken another giant step with the emergence of computer-assisted WSI analysis. To overcome challenges related to optimizing speed and accuracy, numerous statistical manipulations and algorithms have been generated adapted, and adopted to enhance the detection, quantification, and characterization of pathology. In this chapter, both the histories and current state of digital pathology and WSI analysis are reviewed, as well as the challenges that remain to optimize their use. It is clear that the potential of digital pathology is almost boundless, but that much work remains to be done.

Keywords Digital pathology · Image analysis · Histological analysis · Object recognition

4.1 Current Technology and Challenges

The traditional histological/pathological model, which continues to be used as the gold standard, consists of a single operator, typically a pathologist, visually examining a slide looking for specific tissue characteristics, such as atypical cells or nuclei, the presence of inflammatory cells, cell invasion across tissue barriers, or evidence of tissue necrosis. This process is aided by the addition of various stains but is restricted by the lack of objectivity and reproducibility, the small number of characteristics that the human eye can detect within a reasonable period of time, and the considerable variability that exists between operators [1], as well as the examiner's inability to assess any more than the small sampled sections of a slide that fall within single visual fields. Moreover, it is extremely inefficient from a time management perspective. Not only are human eyes limited in the number of characteristics they can seek in a given visual field at any given time, they also often must cipher through volumes of normal tissue to identify any area with pathology. For example, of all the prostate biopsies performed in the USA to detect malignancy, only 20 % reveal any clinically relevant pathology [2], and this low percentage persists even in selected patients with abnormal digital prostate examinations and increased serum markers such as prostate-specific antigen [3]. Similarly, of the approximately one million breast biopsies performed each year in the USA, only between 20 and 30 % demonstrate any evidence of malignancy [4]. What these numbers mean is that, even in highly selected patients, pathologists are spending the vast majority of their time assessing normal tissue.

In an attempt to more effectively and efficiently utilize digital whole slide images (WSIs), over time, there has been a huge push toward *computer-assisted diagnosis* and *computer image analysis*, conjoined concepts that hearken back to the initial use of digital mammography in the early 1990s [5], a practice that itself has evolved to widespread use for the clinical detection of breast cancer across the USA [6]. In particular, over the past decade, the use of computers to assist in clinical diagnosis has blossomed into the evaluation of WSI, where it is increasingly allowing for the objective, rapid, and reproducible evaluation of numerous cellular and extracellular characteristics. Today, in excess of one hundred different cellular and extracellular characteristics can be assessed almost simultaneously through parallelization. The small individual units are generally referred to as *superpixels* or sometimes image objects. They are in effect polygonal parts of a digital image that are larger than a normal pixel and rendered in the same color and brightness. Moreover, WSI analysis allows for comparison of all these characteristics within a given superpixel against neighboring superpixels. To achieve this, a complex series of steps must be undertaken to convert visual data to digital and then to statistically interpretable numerical data, many of them using mathematical models and algorithms that allow for specific quantification and analyses. One component of this process is that stains can be both detected and quantified [7, 8]. This is accomplished using recent innovations such as

- *automated histopathology pattern recognition* [9]
- *color enhancement and standardization* techniques [10–12]
- *color content analysis* that allows for the detection and quantification of histochemical stains [13]
- *image microarrays* (IMA) and *multiplexed biomarker testing*

This all is done, so several tissue characteristics, biomarkers, or stains can be sought and detected on the same slide, thereby replacing the tedious-to-make and difficult-to-maintain cell blocks of traditional microscopy [14, 15].

Among numerous other uses, these algorithms allow for the (semi-)automatic detection and characterization of cancerous cells [16], potentially replacing the fastidious manual searches of pathologists that, as stated earlier, may detect nothing but normal tissue up to 80 % of the time. They also are being utilized to characterize cancers, guide their treatment, and predict prognosis. For example, automated image analysis of routine histological sections is now being used to detect and quantify the expression of human epidermal growth factor receptor (HER2) in breast cancer, since over-expression is associated with an increased risk of recurrence and poor outcomes and predicts responsiveness to trastuzumab, a monoclonal antibody that targets the HER2/neu receptor [17]. Similarly, immunohistochemistry techniques have been combined with digital pattern recognition-based image analysis to identify a specific phenotype of colorectal cancer [18]. This is but scratching the surface, however. Given the tremendous number of diseases and the even greater number of histological markers of disease involving nuclei, cytoplasm, and cell membranes (for example, the detection of breast cancer cells protein receptors such as ER, PR, HER2, Ki-67, and P53), as well as extracellular substrate, there continues to be a huge call for improved informatics tools to ease the massive-scale visualization and analysis of data.

Nowadays, multipurpose tools and programming libraries such as Openslide [19, 20] and Bio-formats [21] aim to assist users and developers with reading an increasing number of WSI formats. Once the WSI is opened and accessible, another major challenge is to optimize the speed of image analysis algorithms performed on each and every region of interest in the WSI. The speed issue is critical because of the tremendous volume of slides that is generated in current clinical practice. For example, Isaacs et al. [22] reported that their facility processed roughly 15,000 slides daily. If the average per-image processing time of 60–90 s reported at Massachusetts General Hospital [23] is a reflection of processing elsewhere, any facility averaging 15,000 images per day would require between 10 and 15 images be processed continuously, 24/7/365, to keep up with demands.

As described in the previous section, concerns regarding image processing speed have led to a proliferation of WSI management systems designed to enhance the capture, storage, retrieval, and dissemination of virtual slides and specimens [24–27]. Moreover, cloud-based platforms such as Histobox (https://www.histobox.com) and Simagis (http://www.simagis.com) are increasingly being used to perform high-demand whole slide imaging tasks on servers other than the computers that pathologists use. However, markedly enhancing the speed of WSI diagnostics via the use of computer-assisted analysis is central to any attempts to significantly reduce processing times further. Moreover, accuracy must be maintained, if not augmented. To achieve both of these ends, speed of analysis and accuracy of results, numerous image algorithms are already being utilized on WSI, some of which starts even before capturing the image is complete.

As the name implies, *image preprocessing* is one of the earliest steps and, in fact, consists of several steps. One essential component is the normalization of color and degree of illumination. This step is required because histopathological assessment invariably relies on the application of various dyes and immunofluorescent stains and counterstains to identify specific cellular and extracellular components and markers of disease, and this application is never entirely homogeneous. Similarly, image scanning is typically non-uniform. To reduce image-to-image variation and the blurring of clear thresholds, these discrepancies can be minimized in a number of ways that include using calibration targets, estimating the illumination pattern from a series of images by fitting polynomial surfaces, and utilizing image gradients estimated in CEI-LUV color space [28–33]. Another strategy involves matching histograms of the images using a variety of specialized software packages that have been developed to adjust for both spectral and spatial illumination [34].

A second essential component of image preprocessing is compensating for tissue auto-fluorescence, an issue that arises in various scenarios, but notably in retrospective studies involving formalin-fixed, paraffin-embedded tissue sections [2]. For this, a multi-step algorithm involving two-stage tissue dye application and several mathematical transformations has been developed [29, 35, 36]. The end result is an image in which areas of high auto-fluorescence, such as blood cells and fat, are removed, allowing for a much clearer depiction of the disease marker(s) or other tissue characteristics being sought and, hence, for their detection, enumeration, and characterization.

After image preprocessing, a second essential step in the detection of pathology for computer-assisted diagnosis is to automatically detect certain histological structures, starting with larger tissue structures like the mucosal layer in the colon, proceeding to tissue cells and migratory cells like leukocytes and lymphocytes, and then to smaller intracellular structures like mitochondria and nuclei; and to be able to determine their number, size, shape, and other morphological features [2]. There is a problem with the standard for identification and quantitation. A mitochondrion in cross section looks very different from a mitochondrion in longitudinal section. This is even more so if sliced obliquely. Also, variations in the location of subcellular components in the z-axis generate variations in size for same-sized objects. As stated above, this all must be accurate, a goal that still warrants considerable work for certain structures and settings. To date, for example, count accuracy rates have varied from as low as 60 % to as high as 98 %, depending upon the methods used, the tissue being studied, and the specific feature being counted (e.g., nuclei versus mitoses) [37–41].

Segmentation is one process by which specific cytological structures are identified and can be restricted to specific structures like nuclei or mitochondria [42, 43], or be more global to include entire cells or tissues [2, 44], whereby either different algorithms are utilized to identify different structures or the same algorithm is used in different modes. Similarly, structures can be identified by seeking specific markers within them, or via computational methods, like Hessian matrix Eigenvalues for curvature to distinguish between ridge-like membrane structures and more amorphous and rounded (blob-like) nuclear structures [2]. For most forms of cancer, for example, it is critical to delineate epithelial from stromal and connective tissue, which can be accomplished by enumerating specific epithelial cell markers. For example, Sharangpani et al. [45] have used imaging algorithms that incorporated both colorimetric (RGB) and intensity (gray scale) determinations to quantify estrogen and progesterone receptor immune-reactivity in human breast cancer tissue.

Another step, once basic structures are identified, is *feature extraction*, which is generically the process of simplifying the resources required to accurately describe a large set of data. When analyzing complex data, one major challenge stems from the number of variables involved. Analysis involving a large number of variables generally requires either extensive memory and computational power or some classification algorithm that over-fits the training sample and generalizes poorly to new samples. With feature extraction, variable combinations are generated to circumvent

4.1 Current Technology and Challenges

this challenge. In WSI analysis, this involves extracting specific object-level features of identified structures, like their area, various incorporated shapes (e.g., elliptical, convex), center of mass, optical density, fractal dimension, and image band intensity, among many others. Structural information can be further categorized graphically by examining spatially related features to define a large set of topological elements and thereby identify tissue organization, including the clustering of cells and tissue characteristics around such clusters, like the number of nodes, edges, triangles and k-walks, spectral radius, Eigen exponent, roundness factor, and homogeneity. Such a stereological assessment of structures is associated with tremendous inter-rater variability when performed manually [46]. Digitally, cell graphs can be constructed in both two and three dimensions, and the resulting models then used for a variety of purposes such as differentiating different cell types within a given tissue by modeling the extracellular matrix [47] and determining cancer grade [48].

Multi-scale feature extraction mimics the human approach to visualizing a slide, which typically entails adjusting resolution to view different characteristics. For example, at low resolution, the overall topology of the slide is seen; at medium resolution, larger structures like nuclei can be detected; and at high resolution, the morphology of more specific histological structures like nucleoli, mitochondria, and endoplasmic reticulum can be delineated [2]. This same approach can be used digitally, starting with the lowest resolution and progressing to higher levels of resolution for more detailed information for analysis [49, 50]. To achieve this, Sertel et al. decomposed images into multi-resolution representations using a Gaussian pyramid. They followed this with sequential color-space conversion and feature construction and then by feature extraction and selection at each resolution level. Classification labels (e.g., differentiated vs. undifferentiated) then were assigned to each image tile and the tiles combined to form an overall classification map [2]. Using this approach, Doyle et al. [51] were able to accurately detect areas of malignancy in prostate tissue samples.

Algorithms also have been developed, modified, or adopted from other applications for a number of other purposes including

- *feature selection*—the process of reducing the number of variables being analyzed by identifying those features that are most diagnostically relevant [52–60];
- *dimensionality reduction*—which similarly reduces the number of variables being considered using statistical tools such as *principal component analysis* [61], *linear discriminant analysis* [62], and *independent component analysis* [63] to handle especially large numbers of variables [64–67];
- *manifold learning*—which is one of a large number of statistical manipulations designed to handle data that require more than two or even three dimensions to be represented, utilizing the assumptions that (1) the data of interest lie on an embedded nonlinear manifold within a higher dimensional space but also that (2) the manifold can be reduced, allowing for the data to be visualized in a lower dimensional space.

Such algorithms include graph embedding constructs, Gaussian process latent variable models, and diffusion maps [68–72], among others.

All of the above-mentioned tools have been used outside of histopathology for other types of image, in medicine most often radiographic, but also with such functions as facial recognition programs [73]. Where histopathology tends to differ, in terms of its relevant information, is in the tremendous density of data that must be detected and analyzed; this is where various classification and subcellular quantification tools become most useful. Multiple classifier and learning ensemble systems work on the premise that the accuracy of identification is accentuated by using multiple instead of single classifiers, both by limiting bias and reducing the high degree of variance that sometimes exists with a single model [2]. As with many of the previously mentioned procedures, multiple classifier and learning ensemble systems rely on a variety of statistical manipulations such as principal component and linear discriminant analysis, but also on techniques such as the kernel function, which allows for data to be projected into high-dimensional space. Numerous examples exist of these techniques being used to accurately diagnose a variety of cancerous lesions, including prostate cancer [70, 74–76], adenocarcinoma of the colon [77, 78], meningioma [79], malignant mesothelioma [80], breast cancer [80, 81], and lung cancer [82].

Even with all of these advancements, and with many more on the way, another perhaps final major obstacle that remains in the way of digital pathology's widespread adoption is the lack of standardization that exists in the field. In light of this, national and international efforts are being undertaken to standardize each stage, orchestrated by organizations such as the International Academy of Digital Pathology, the College of American Pathologists' Diagnostic Intelligence and Health Information (DIHIT) Committee, and EURO-TELEPATH, the primary telepathology network in Europe [83–86]. Standardization is critical not only for diagnostics, but also given the widespread acceptance digital pathology is now receiving as an educational tool [86–91]. Its advantages in terms of creating a permanent, easily accessible and readily transferrable system of pathology slide and specimen archiving also are clear.

4.2 Current State of Digital Pathology and WSI Analysis

It is clear that digital pathology and WSI analysis are carving their place as invaluable research tools. However, there also is evidence that this emerging field is becoming of increasing value within the context of clinical practice. Several studies have now been published comparing traditional light microscopy with whole slide imaging. In one such study, automated image analysis was discovered to be 95 % accurate identifying low-grade astrocytoma, (WHO grade II), 91 % accurate identifying high-grade (WHO grades III and IV), and 83 % accurate identifying what were termed intermediate grade lesions (grade II/III) [92]; moreover, relatively minor modifications increased overall accuracy to almost 98 % [93]. Meanwhile, Ho et al. [94] performed a pilot retrospective validation study to test for quality assurance (QA) in an automated high-speed WSI system being utilized for surgical genitourinary

4.2 Current State of Digital Pathology and WSI Analysis

cases. In this study, 24 full cases (including 47 surgical parts and 391 slides) were independently reviewed with traditional microscopy and whole slide digital images, with diagnostic discrepancies evaluated by a pathology consensus committee. In the end, participating pathologists claimed that the traditional and WSI methods were comparable for case review and reported no differences in perceived case complexity or diagnostic confidence between the methods. A total of four clinically insignificant discrepancies were noted, two from glass slides and two from WSI review. Ultimately, there was consensus that automated WSI is a viable potential modality for surgical pathology QA, especially in multi-facility health systems that would like to establish inter-facility QA. Moreover, participants felt that major issues limiting the implementation of WSI-based QA did not involve image acquisition or quality, but rather image management issues such as the pathologist's interface, the hospital network, and integration with the laboratory information system [94]. In yet another study, both the sensitivity and specificity of three-dimensional WSI were found to be 95 %, comparable to visual microscopy [95].

In another small validation study, three pathologists came to consensus diagnoses for 25 cases that included biopsies of skin, bladder, urethra, prostate, and kidney, and no significant discrepancies were identified between consensus reached with virtual (WSI) versus visual slides [96]. Fine et al. performed a similar validation study with five pathologists and 31 prostate biopsy cases, and there was only one case in which a significant discrepancy arose. The overall level of agreement ($\kappa = 0.817$) was considered excellent [97]. Finally, in a multi-site study conducted at the Mayo Clinic, 520 formalin-fixed breast tissue specimens were assayed at three clinical sites for estrogen and progesterone receptors (260 each) [98]. At each participating site, three pathologists performed a blinded reading of the glass slides using their microscopes initially and later using digital images on a computer monitor, assessing the percentage and average staining intensity of positive nuclei. Comparable percentages of agreement were obtained for manual microscopy and manual digital slide reading, ranging between 83.8 and 99.0 % for the manual technique and from 76.3 to 100.0 % with the monitor, depending upon what characteristic was being assessed.

In terms of the effectiveness and efficiency of uploading digital images into a designated central server for use by several facilities in a network, of 26.966 gross images retrospectively reviewed out of 9.733 cases that were automatically uploaded over a three-year period onto a networked image server serving 20 hospitals, only 45 images failed the automatic upload and had to be uploaded manually [25].

As such, it is clear that many of the obstacles initially envisioned for virtual pathology systems have since been addressed and that the value and potential uses of digital pathology are expanding exponentially, in parallel with advances in technology [83, 88, 99–103].

The question arises: What further challenges remain? Besides convincing pathologists to adopt the newer systems over traditional methods, for reasons that include lack of familiarity and adequate training and concerns over costs and the future of pathologists themselves (Are they to be replaced by machines?) [22, 89, 94, 104–106], challenges also continue to exist over the technical logistics of WSI analysis itself. However, in this rapidly evolving field, potential solutions to overcoming these challenges are seemingly being generated every day.

The next chapter provides specific use cases demonstrating how digital pathology, whole slide imaging, and image analysis can be applied in various clinical and research scenarios.

4.3 Toward In Silico Pathology

Image analysis is a big enough topic to warrant its own chapter. It is no surprise that this field has taken off so quickly, as many *in silico* techniques can be brought in from other specialties, including but not limited to medical imaging, bioinformatics, and engineering.

One remarkable observation is that image analysis in WSI is often still remarkably primitive. Many protocols are still based on color separation techniques, and object detection is still a relatively new concept that is just now becoming mainstream. On the other hand, more advanced algorithms usually mean longer computation times. It would appear then that this is at least one impediment to a major breakthrough: The computer (for now) still needs more time than a trained pathologist to come to a diagnosis.

In the next chapter, we will discuss a number of specific implementations (case studies).

References

1. Fanshawe, T.R., Lynch, A.G., Ellis, I.O., Green, A.R., Hanka, R.: Assessing agreement between multiple raters with missing rating information, applied to breast cancer tumour grading. PLoS ONE **3**, e2925 (2008)
2. Gurcan, M.N., Boucheron, L., Can, A., et al.: Histopathological image analysis: a review. IEEE Rev. Biomed. Eng. **2**, 141–171 (2009)
3. Roychowdhury, A., Basu, S., Bandyapadhyay, A., Bhattacharya, P., Mitra, R.B.: Kappa statistics in the screening of malignancy of prostate. J. Indian Med. Assoc. **109**, 786–789 (2011)
4. Core-Needle Biopsy for Breast Abnormalities: Clinician's Guide. U.S. Department of Health and Human Services (2010)
5. Mendez, A.J., Tahoces, P.G., Lado, M.J., Souto, M., Vidal, J.J.: Computer-aided diagnosis: automatic detection of malignant masses in digitized mammograms. Med. Phys. **25**, 957–964 (1998)
6. Tang, J., Rangayyan, R.M., Xu, J., El Naqa, I., Yang, Y.: Computer-aided detection and diagnosis of breast cancer with mammography: recent advances. IEEE Trans. Inf. Technol. Biomed. **13**, 236–251 (2009)
7. Varga, V.S., Ficsor, L., Kamaras, V., et al.: Automated multichannel fluorescent whole slide imaging and its application for cytometry. Cytometry A. **75**, 1020–1030 (2009)
8. Martina, J.D., Simmons, C., Jukic, D.M.: High-definition hematoxylin and eosin staining in a transition to digital pathology. J. Pathol. Inform. **2**, 45 (2011)
9. Webster, J.D., Michalowski, A.M., Dwyer, J.E., et al.: Investigation into diagnostic agreement using automated computer-assisted histopathology pattern recognition image analysis. J. Pathol. Inform. **3**, 18 (2012)

10. Bautista, P., Yagi, Y.: Digital simulation of staining in histopathology multispectral images: enhancement and linear transformation of spectral transmittance. J. Biomed. Opt. **17** (2012)
11. Tani, S.: Color standardization system implementing estimation method for absorption spectra of dye. Anal. Cell. Pathol. **34**, 180 (2013)
12. Yagi, Y.: Color standardization and optimization in whole slide imaging. Diagn. Pathol. **6**, S15 (2011)
13. Keller, B., Chen, W., Gavrielides, M.A.: Quantitative assessment and classification of tissue-based biomarker expression with color content analysis. Arch. Pathol. Lab. Med. **136**, 539–550 (2012)
14. Nederlof, M., Watanabe, S., Burnip, B., Taylor, D.L., Critchley-Thorne, R.: High-throughput profiling of tissue and tissue model microarrays: combined transmitted light and 3-color fluorescence digital pathology. J. Pathol. Inform. **2**, 50 (2011)
15. Hipp, J., Cheng, J., Pantanowitz, L., et al.: Image microarrays (IMA): digital pathology's missing tool. J. Pathol. Inform. **2**, 47 (2011)
16. Feldman, M.D.: Beyond morphology: whole slide imaging, computer-aided detection, and other techniques. Arch. Pathol. Lab. Med. **132**, 758–763 (2008)
17. Nanda, R.: Targeting the human epidermal growth factor receptor 2 (HER2) in the treatment of breast cancer: recent advances and future directions. Rev. Recent Clin. Trials **2**, 111–116 (2007)
18. Angell, H.K., Gray, N., Womack, C., et al.: Digital pattern recognition-based image analysis quantifies immune infiltrates in distinct tissue regions of colorectal cancer and identifies a metastatic phenotype. Br. J. Cancer **109**, 1618–1624 (2013)
19. Goode, A., Gilbert, G., Harkes, J., Jukic, D., Satyanarayanan, M.: OpenSlide: A vendor-neutral software foundation for digital pathology. J. Pathol. Inform. **4**, 27 (2013)
20. Open Slide: National Institutes of Health, Clinical and Translational Science Institute, University of Pittsburgh (2014)
21. Bioformats: Laboratory for Optical and Computational Instrumentation (2014)
22. Isaacs, M., Lennerz, J.K., Yates, S., et al.: Implementation of whole slide imaging in surgical pathology: a value added approach. J. Pathol. Inform. **2**, 39 (2011)
23. McClintock, D.S., Lee, R.E., Gilbertson, J.R.: Using computerized workflow simulations to assess the feasibility of Whole Slide Imaging full adoption in a high volume histology laboratory. Anal. Cell. Pathol. **34**, 182–184 (2013)
24. Krupinski, E.A.: Optimizing the pathology workstation "cockpit": challenges and solutions. J. Pathol. Inform. **1**, 19 (2010)
25. Amin, M., Sharma, G., Parwani, A.V., et al.: Integration of digital gross pathology images for enterprise-wide access. J. Pathol. Inform. **3**, 10 (2012)
26. Wang, F., Oh, T.W., Vergara-Niedermayr, C., Kurc, T., Saltz, J.: Managing and querying whole slide images. In: Proceedings of SPIE, vol. 8319(pii), pp. 83190J, 16 Feb 2012
27. Wang, Y., Williamson, K.E., Kelly, P.J., James, J.A., Hamilton, P.W.: SurfaceSlide: a multi-touch digital pathology platform. PLoS ONE **7**, e30783 (2012)
28. Gurcan, M.N., Boucheron, L., Can, A., et al.: Histopathological image analysis: a review. IEEE Rev. Biomed. Eng. **2**, 141–171 (2009)
29. Can, A., Bello, M., Cline, H.C., Tao, X., Ginty, F., Sood, A., Gerdes, M., Montalto, M.: Multimodal imaging of histological tissue sections. In: 5th IEEE International Symposium on Biomedical Imaging: From Nano to Macro, pp. 288–291 (2008)
30. Yang, L., Meer, P., Foran, D.J.: Unsupervised segmentation based on robust estimation and color active contour models. IEEE Trans. Inf. Technol. Biomed. **9**, 475–486 (2005)
31. Wang, Y.Y., Chang, S.C., Wu, L.W., Tsai, S.T., Sun, Y.N.: A color-based approach for automated segmentation in tumor tissue classification. Conf. Proc. IEEE Eng. Med. Biol. Soc. 6577–6580 (2007)
32. Sun, Y.N., Wang, Y.Y., Chang, S.C., Wu, L.W., Tsai, S.T.: Color-based tumor tissue segmentation for the automated estimation of oral cancer parameters. Microsc. Res. Tech. **73**, 5–13 (2010)
33. Kayser, G., Kayser, K.: Quantitative pathology in virtual microscopy: history, applications, perspectives. Acta Histochem. **115**, 527–532 (2013)

34. Gurcan, M.N., Boucheron, L., Can, A., et al.: Histopathological image analysis: a review. IEEE Rev. Biomed. Eng. **2**, 141–171 (2009)
35. Bello, M., Can, A., Tao, X.: Accurate registration and failure detection in tissue micro array images. In: 5th IEEE International Symposium Biomedical Imaging: From Nano to Macro, pp. 368–371 (2008)
36. Narasimha-Iyer, H., Can, A., Roysam, B., et al.: Robust detection and classification of longitudinal changes in color retinal fundus images for monitoring diabetic retinopathy. IEEE Trans. Biomed. Eng. **53**, 1084–1098 (2006)
37. Bibbo, M., Kim, D.H., Pfeifer, T., et al.: Histometric features for the grading of prostatic carcinoma. Anal. Quant. Cytol. Histol. **13**, 61–68 (1991)
38. Belein, J.A., Baak, J.P., Van Diest, P.J., van Ginkel, A.H.: Counting mitoses by image processing in Feulgen stained breast cancer sections: the influence of resolution. Cytometry **28**, 135–140 (1997)
39. Markiewicz, T., Osowski, S., Patera, J., Kozlowski, W.: Image processing for accurate cell recognition and count on histologic slides. Anal. Quant. Cytol. Histol. **28**, 281–291 (2006)
40. Kim, Y.L., Romeike, B.F., Uszkoreit, J., Feiden, W.: Automated nuclear segmentation in the determination of the Ki-67 labeling index in meningiomas. Clin. Neuropathol. **25**, 67–73 (2006)
41. Sont, J.K., De Boer, W.I., van Schadewijk, W.A., et al.: Fully automated assessment of inflammatory cell counts and cytokine expression in bronchial tissue. Am. J. Respir. Crit. Care Med. **167**, 1503 (2003)
42. Brock, R., Hink, M.A., Jovin, T.M.: Fluorescence correlation microscopy of cells in the presence of autofluorescence. Biophys. J. **75**, 2547–2557 (2014)
43. Gerencser, A.A., Adam-Vizi, V.: Selective, high-resolution fluorescence imaging of mitochondrial Ca^{2+} concentration. Cell Calcium **30**, 311–321 (2001)
44. Can, A., Bello, M., Cline, H.E., Tao, X., Ginty, F., Sood, A., Gerdes, M., Montalto, M.: Multimodal imaging of histological tissue sections. In: 5th IEEE International Symposium Biomedical Imaging: From Nano to Macro 2008, pp. 288–291 (2008)
45. Sharangpani, G.M., Joshi, A.S., Porter, K., et al.: Semi-automated imaging system to quantitate estrogen and progesterone receptor immunoreactivity in human breast cancer. J. Microsc. **226**, 244–255 (2007)
46. Gundersen, H.J., Osterby, R.: Optimizing sampling efficiency of stereological studies in biology: or 'do more less well!'. J. Microsc. **121**, 65–73 (1981)
47. Bilgin, C.C., Bullough, P., Plopper, G.E., Yener, B.: ECM-Aware Cell-Graph mining for bone tissue modeling and classification. Data Min. Knowl. Discov. **20**, 416–438 (2009)
48. Doyle, S., Hwang, M., Shah, K., et al.: Automated grading of prostate cancer using architectural and textural image features. IEEE Explore 1284–1287 (2007)
49. Sertel, O., Kong, J., Shimada, H., et al.: Computer-aided prognosis of neuroblastoma on whole-slide images: classification of stromal development. Pattern Recognit. **42**, 1093–1103 (2009)
50. Sertel, O., Kong, J., Shimada, H., et al.: Computer-aided prognosis of neuroblastoma on whole-slide images: classifying grade of neuroblastic differentiation. Pattern Recognit. **42**, 1080–1192 (2009)
51. Doyle, S., Madabhushi, A., Feldman, M., Tomaszeweski, J.: A boosting cascade for automated detection of prostate cancer from digitized histology. Med. Image Comput. Comput. Assist. Interv. **9**, 504–511 (2006)
52. Pudil, P., Novovicvova, J., Kittler, J.: Floating search methods in feature selection. Pattern Recogn. Lett. **15**, 1119–1125 (1994)
53. Jain, A., Zongker, D.: Feature selection: evaluation, application, and small sample performance. IEEE Trans. Pattern Anal. Mach. Intell. **19**, 153–158 (1997)
54. Freund, Y., Shapire, R.E.: A decision-theoretic generalization of on-line learning and an application to boosting. J. Comp. Syst. Sci. **55**, 119–139 (1997)
55. Perkins, S., Lacker, K., Theiler, J.: Fast, incremental feature selection by gradient descent in function space. J. Mach. Learn. Res. **3**, 1333–1356 (2003)
56. Qureshi, H., Sertel, O., Rajpoot, N., Wilson, R., Gurcan, M.N.: Adaptive discriminant wavelet packet transform and local binary patterns for meningioma subtype classification.

In: Medical Image Computing and Computer-Assisted Intervention—MICCAI 2008, pp. 196–204
57. Pudil, P., Novovivcova, J.: Novel methods for feature subset selection with respect to problem knowledge. In: Feature Extraction, Construction and Selection, p. 101 (1998)
58. Samet, H.: Foundations of Multidimensional and Metric Data Structures. Morgan Kaufmann, Los Altos (2006)
59. Ding, C., He, X., Zha, H., Simon, H.D.: Adaptive dimension reduction for clustering high dimensional data. In: International Conference on Data Mining (2002)
60. Lu, H., Plataniotis, K.N., Venetsanopoulos, A.N.: A survey of multilinear subspace learning for tensor data. IEEE Rev. Biomed. Eng. **2**, 171 (2009)
61. Jolliffe, I.: Principal Component Analysis, 2nd edn. Springer, Berlin (2002)
62. Martinez, A., Kak, A.: PCA versus LDA. IEEE Trans. Pattern Anal. Mach. Intell. **23**, 228–233 (2001)
63. Chawla, N.V., Bowyer, K.W.: Designing Multiple Classifier Systems for Face Recognition. Department of Computer Science and Engineering, University of Notre Dame (2014)
64. Hu, H., Zahorian, S.A.: Dimensionality Reduction Methods for HMM Phonetic Recognition. Department of Electrical and Computer Engineering, Binghamton University (2010)
65. Shaw, B., Jebara, T.: Structure preserving embedding. In: Proceedings of the 26th Annual International Conference on Machine Learning—ICML'09. 1, 2009
66. Bingham, E., Mannila, H.: Random projection in dimensionality reduction. In: Proceedings of the Seventh ACM SIGKDD International Conference on Knowledge Discovery and Data Mining—KDD'01. 245, 2001
67. Roweis, S.T., Saul, L.K.: Nonlinear dimensionality reduction by locally linear embedding. Science **290**, 2323–2326 (2000)
68. Gao, X., Wang, X., Tao, D., Li, X.: Supervised Gaussian process latent variable model for dimensionality reduction. IEEE Trans. Syst. Man Cybern. B Cybern. **41**, 425–434 (2011)
69. Madabhushi, A., Doyle, S., Lee, J.H., et al.: Integrated diagnostics: a conceptual framework with examples. Clin. Chem. Lab. Med. **48**, 998 (2010)
70. Doyle, S., Hwang, M., Shah, K., Madabhushi, A., Feldman, M., Tomaszewski, J.: Automated grading of prostate cancer using architectural and textural image features. In: 4th IEEE International Symposium on Biomedical Imaging: From Nano to Macro, 2007. ISBI 2007, pp. 1284–1287
71. Rajpoot, N., Mohammad, A., Bhalerao, A.: Unsupervised learning of shape manifolds. In: Proceedings of the British Machine Vision Conference 2007 (2014)
72. Coifman, R., Lafon, S., Lee, A., Maggioni, M., Nadler, B., Warner, F., Zucker, S.: Geometric diffusions as a tool for harmonic analysis and structure definition of data: diffusion maps. In: Proceedings of the National Academy of Sciences, pp. 7426–7431 (2005)
73. Chawla, N.V., Bowyer, K.W.: Designing Multiple Classifier Systems for Face Recognition. Department of Computer Science and Engineering, University of Notre Dame (2014)
74. Doyle, S., Rodriguez, C., Madabhushi, A., Tomaszewski, J., Feldman, M.: Detecting prostatic adenocarcinoma from digitized histology using a multi-scale, hierarchical classification approach. In: IEEE Engineering in Medicine and Biology Conference, pp. 4759–4762 (2014)
75. Jafari-Khouzani, K., Soltanian-Zadeh, H.: Multiwavelet grading of pathological images of prostate. IEEE Trans. Biomed. Eng. **50**, 697–704 (2003)
76. Tabesh, A., Teverovskiy, M., Pang, H.Y., et al.: Multifeature prostate cancer diagnosis and Gleason grading of histological images. IEEE Trans. Med. Imaging **26**, 1366–1378 (2007)
77. Rajpoot, K., Rajpoot, N.: Optimization for hyperspectral colon tissue cell classification. In: Medical Image Computing and Computer-Assisted Intervention. MICCAI-2004, pp. 829–837 (2004)
78. Esgiar, A.N., Naguib, R.N., Sharif, B.S., Bennett, M.K., Murray, A.: Microscopic image analysis for quantitative measurement and feature identification of normal and cancerous colonic mucosa. IEEE Trans. Inf. Technol. Biomed. **2**, 197–203 (1998)
79. Qureshi, H., Sertel, O., Rajpoot, N., Wilson, R., Gurcan, M.N.: Adaptive discriminant wavelet packet transform and local binary patterns for meningioma subtype classification. Med. Image Comput. Comput. Assist. Interv. **11**, 196–204 (2008)

80. van de Wouwer, G., Weyn, B., Scheunders, P., et al.: Wavelets as chromatin texture descriptors for the automated identification of neoplastic nuclei. J. Microsc. **197**, 25–35 (2000)
81. Winzer, K.J., Bellach, J., Hufnagl, P.: Long-term analysis to objectify the tumour grading by means of automated microscopic image analysis of the nucleolar organizer regions (AgNORs) in the case of breast carcinoma. Diagn. Pathol. **8**, 56 (2013). doi: 10.1186/1746-1596-8-56
82. Weyn, B., van de Wouwer, G., van Daele, A., et al.: Automated breast tumor diagnosis and grading based on wavelet chromatin texture description. Cytometry **33**, 32–40 (1998)
83. Garcia Rojo, M.: State of the art and trends for digital pathology. Stud. Health Technol. Inform. **179**, 15–28 (2012)
84. Evans, A., Sinard, J.H., Fatheree, L.A., Henricks, W.H., Carter, A.B., Contis, L., et al.: Validating whole slide imaging for diagnostic purposes in pathology: recommendations of the College of American Pathologists (CAP) pathology and laboratory quality centre. Anal. Cell. Pathol. **34**, 174 (2011)
85. Singh, R., Chubb, L., Pantanowitz, L., Parwani, A.: Standardization in digital pathology: Supplement 145 of the DICOM standards. J. Pathol. Inform. **2**, 23 (2011)
86. Yagi, Y., Rojo, M.G., Kayser, K., et al.: The first congress of the International Academy of Digital Pathology: digital pathology comes of age. Anal. Cell. Pathol. (AMST) **35**, 1–2 (2012)
87. Huisman, A.: Digital pathology for education. Stud. Health Technol. Inform. **179**, 68–71 (2012)
88. Wilbur, D.C.: Digital cytology: current state of the art and prospects for the future. Acta Cytol. **55**, 227–238 (2011)
89. Tsuchihasi, Y.: Expanding application of digital pathology in Japan—from education, telepathology to autodiagnosis. Diagn. Pathol. **6**, S19 (2011)
90. Hamilton, P.W., Wang, Y., McCullough, S.J.: Virtual microscopy and digital pathology in training and education. APMIS **120**, 305–315 (2012)
91. Schwartz, J.: Expanding the lab's reach with digital pathology. MLO Med. Lab. Obs. **43**, 41 (2011)
92. Glotsos, D., Tohka, J., Ravazoula, P., Cavouras, D., Nikifordis, G.: Automated diagnosis of brain tumours astrocytomas using probabilistic neural network clustering and support vector machines. Int. J. Neural Syst. **15**, 1–11 (2005)
93. Glotsos, D., Kalatzis, I., Spyridonos, P., et al.: Improving accuracy in astrocytomas grading by integrating a robust least squares mapping driven support vector machine classifier into a two level grade classification scheme. Comput. Methods Programs Biomed. **90**, 251–261 (2008)
94. Ho, J., Parwani, A., Jukic, D.M., et al.: Use of whole slide imaging in surgical pathology quality assurance: design and pilot validation studies. Hum. Pathol. **37**, 322–331 (2006)
95. Kalinski, T., Zwonitzer, R., Sel, S., et al.: Virtual 3D microscopy using multiplane whole slide images in diagnostic pathology. Am. J. Clin. Pathol. **130**, 259–264 (2008)
96. Gilbertson, J.R., Ho, J., Anthony, L., et al.: Primary histologic diagnosis using automated whole slide imaging: a validation study. BMC Clin. Pathol. **27**, 4 (2006)
97. Fine, J.L., Grzybicki, D.M., Silowash, R., et al.: Evaluation of whole slide image immunohistochemistry interpretation in challenging prostate needle biopsies. Hum. Pathol. **39**, 564–572 (2008)
98. Nassar, A., Cohen, C., Agersborg, S.S., et al.: A multisite performance study comparing the reading of immunohistochemical slides on a computer monitor with conventional manual microscopy for estrogen and progesterone receptor analysis. Am. J. Clin. Pathol. **135**, 461–467 (2011)
99. Pantanowitz, L.: Digital images and the future of digital pathology. J. Pathol. Inform. **10**, 1 (2010)
100. Pantanowicz, L., Szymas, J., Yagi, Y., Wilbur, D.: Whole slide imaging for educational purposes. J. Pathol. Inform. **3** (2012)

References

101. Al-Janabi, S., Huisman, A., Van Diest, P.J.: Digital pathology: current status and future perspectives. Histopathology **61**, 1–9 (2012)
102. Hedvat, C.V.: Digital microscopy: past, present, and future. Arch. Pathol. Lab. Med. **134**, 1666–1670 (2010)
103. Pantanowitz, L., Wiley, C.A., Demetris, A., et al.: Experience with multimodality telepathology at the University of Pittsburgh Medical Center. J. Pathol. Inform. **3**, 45 (2013). doi: 10.4103/2153-3539.104907. Epub 20 Dec 2012
104. Dennis, T., Start, R.D., Cross, S.S.: The use of digital imaging, video conferencing, and telepathology in histopathology: a national survey. J. Clin. Pathol. **58**, 254–258 (2005)
105. Johnson, D.E.: NightHawk teleradiology services: a template for pathology? Arch. Pathol. Lab. Med. **132**, 745–747 (2008)
106. Cornish, T.C., Swapp, R.E., Kaplan, K.J.: Whole-slide imaging: routine pathologic diagnosis. Adv. Anat. Pathol. **19**, 152–159 (2012)

Chapter 5
Use Cases

Abstract Previous chapters have demonstrated the evolution of digital pathology, starting as merely a telepathology and educational tool to its more recent use in whole slide image analysis, whereby the computer itself performs diagnostic testing on whole slide images (WSI) to assist pathologists in diagnostic and disease-staging processes. This chapter provides concrete examples of digital pathology at work, ranging from its use aiding in the staging of cancer, to its application as an educational tool at the New York College of Podiatric Medicine (NYCPM), to its adoption as a vital instrument to enhance medical service delivery in developing countries like Egypt and Haiti.

Keywords Digital pathology application · Digital pathology · Telepathology · Biomarker · Primary diagnosis · Second opinion · Pathology education · Quality assurance · Tumor board · Third world · WSI · DP

5.1 Diagnosis and Staging of Disease

5.1.1 Biomarkers

Traditionally, therapeutic decisions in cancer medicine are highly dependent upon well-performed pathological examinations of tumor tissue obtained at biopsy. More recently, the examination of molecular tissue biomarkers has arisen as a means to complement, as opposed to replace, classical histological examinations. These predictive biomarkers are developed during oncology trials with the ultimate goal of predicting a given malignant tumor's response to a specific drug. The concept of personalized medicine represents a transformational event across the fields of oncology, drug trials, cancer diagnostics, and pathology.

The importance of biomarkers is illustrated by the following: On average, chemotherapy is efficacious for only about 5–50 % of cancers, depending on its tissue of origin [1]. Even new and promising immunotherapies only work on a small proportion of cancer patients. Approximately 20–30 % of patients appear to benefit from Food and Drug Administration-approved cytotoxic T-lymphocyte antigen 4 blockade for malignant melanoma [2]. Therefore, it becomes essential to develop biomarkers that can select those patients who have the greatest likelihood of response. Organizations (like clinical and research) must invest (and possibly specialize) in pathological services, with a combined focus on tumor morphology and molecular signatures, while aiming at high-quality, robust molecular assays [3].

5.1.1.1 Digital Analysis of Breast Markers

Breast cancer markers (ER/Her2/Neu) are a good place to start our exploration of the use of whole slide images (WSI), in relation to biomarkers. Image analysis of the estrogen receptor (ER) has been in the literature since the late 1980s. Most early strategies employed a pixel-based approach. The evolution of this field has brought more sophisticated image processing techniques and rules but, with few exceptions, has remained a "bottom–up" approach.

Image processing is typically pixel based and relies on color segmentation and filters. No single-color threshold exists that can correctly classify the nuclei on all slides. It is difficult to find color thresholds that work for a wide range of images. Furthermore, under-segmentation can lead to lost information regarding nuclei shape, which may make it impossible to perform accurate shape analysis downstream.

In contrast, rule-based image analysis relies on blob analysis, as well as rules that combine other (low-level) operations. Challenges of nuclear segmentation are the nuclear segmentation of all nuclei, subsequent correct identification of positive and negative tumor nuclei, and the accurate identification (and filtering) of non-tumor nuclei.

Intra- and inter-slide variability is normal: Nuclei vary in size, shape, and orientation. Tumor morphology and background context vary, as may (background) colors depending on the specific stain used. Positioning of individual cells can lead to its own complexities: Nuclei may overlap or touch each other; and there can be cytoplasm blush and artifacts (non-specific staining). A good segmentation algorithm should be robust to all these variations.

In 2012, at the DPA's annual meeting in Baltimore, USA, Dr. Gerardo Fernandez of Ventana Medical Systems presented recent advances in this field. In his address, he noted that Ventana (which is now a part of Roche) had conducted a clinical trial to assess an object-based learning algorithm to analyze Ki67-, p53-, ER-, and PR-stained samples. The algorithm adopted an object-based supervised learning approach using shape-prior-based nuclei detection.

First, the algorithm was verified on a training slide set. Sixty slides were selected for each marker, reflecting slide variability. Concordance with the manual score was 85–95 %. Next, an FDA clinical validation study was performed, across multiple sites, involving multiple scanners. One hundred and twenty slides were used per marker, and the concordance with manual scores was 85–98 %.

5.1 Diagnosis and Staging of Disease

Eventually, independent validation studies were performed by laboratories (customers). The concordance with manual scores was once again >90 %.

These are really good results and are promising for the future. The challenge is now to adapt this algorithm to work on other bright-field and IF image analysis problems.

5.1.1.2 HistoGeneX and the Evolution to Personalized Medicine

HistoGeneX was founded in 2001 and specializes in advanced histopathological techniques for biomarker discovery, clinical trials, and personalized medicine (http://www.histogenex.com). It combines pathology with tissue biomarkers. The company offers high-quality morphological and molecular pathological services, with ISO-15189/ College of American Pathologists (CAP) and Clinical Laboratory Improvement Amendments (CLIA) accreditation. Therefore, HistoGeneX works under standardized conditions with different standardized processes described in dedicated standard operating procedures (SOPs). Its customers include pharmaceutical companies, diagnostic partners, clinical research organizations, and academic institutions.

Since 2003, HistoGeneX has been involved in several oncology trials and is responsible for tissue biomarker development and validation, as well as good clinical practice/good clinical laboratory practice testing (cancer profiling). For instance, HistoGeneX has played a major role in KRAS testing, leading to the registration of drugs coupled to follow-up of this biomarker [4]. Some of these biomarkers are evaluated with extraction-based methods, while others involve in situ methods. In all situations, the first step is to evaluate the tumor cell content of the biopsy. This is important, in view of the genomic and proteomic heterogeneity that has been discovered in biopsies of solid tumors.

At HistoGeneX, samples are already routinely tested for predictive biomarkers like HER2/neu, anaplastic lymphoma kinase (ALK), epidermal growth factor receptor (EGFR), v-Raf murine sarcoma viral oncogene homolog B1 (BRAF), and v-Ki-ras2 Kirsten rat sarcoma viral oncogene homolog (KRAS). Even so, new tests covering tumor immune responses will be required for immunotherapies, and for other targeted therapies like bevacizumab, which has been shown to affect immunity as well as angiogenesis [5]. Next to its morphological potentials, HistoGeneX established laboratory cores for detailed analysis of molecular signals, including Italian Hospital in Cairo (IHC) IF, flow cytometry, ISH, and RNA/DNA techniques.

Over the years, HistoGeneX has developed, invested, and specialized in pathological services, with a combined focus on tumor morphology and molecular signatures, while aiming at high-quality levels and robust molecular assays. All tumor block analyses start with a certified pathologist evaluating a hematoxylin eosin (HE)-stained slide. The pathologist outlines the regions of interest (e.g., tumor tissue) on a snapshot of the HE-stained slide. This tumor map is used to guide the HistoGeneX imaging scientists through all subsequent imaging analyses. The company maintains stringent optimization and validation policies for the development of new assays. HistoGeneX has acquired several automated stainers (Dako autostainer

Link, Labvision autostainers, Ventana Benchmark XT, Ventana Discovery XT, Ventana Benchmark Ultra). Automated platforms allow for more standardized and controlled assays and are able to cope with large-sample batches. Every newly developed assay at HistoGeneX is consequently tested for accuracy, specificity, and precision. If the accuracy and specificity of one specific target can be ascertained, the precision can be determined by looking at intra- and inter-run variability.

Currently, almost all slides are scanned and permanently stored as WSI. Acquisition of WSI has several advantages. With permanent storage of images of stained slides that are not altered over time (in contrast to staining on real slides), virtual images can be viewed from any computer at any time. Remote viewing also enhances remote consultation, telepathology, and the exchange of image information. Furthermore, WSI are of vital use in the analysis of serial IHC sections and tissue microarrays and are an excellent platform for computer-assisted image analysis.

In addition to reliable and robust assays, uniform qualification of IHC/IF/ISH signals in tumors is of vast importance. By designing and validating an appropriate scoring method, bias can be avoided and results deemed trustworthy. At HistoGeneX, Definiens Architect XD—Tissue Studio is frequently used for nuclear IHC-staining assays in tumors. Carl Zeiss AxioVision is used to measure tissue and tumor areas. Whole slide images in combination with computer-assisted IHC scoring systems offer the opportunity to accurately quantify both staining intensity and the (sub)cellular localization of protein expression in a reproducible and traceable way. Automated analytical approaches provide more detailed quantitative data that can be subjected to more robust statistical analysis than the qualitative or semi-quantitative data that are produced from manual analysis.

5.1.2 Cytology

Cytologies for a unique specimen type are one of the most commonly performed procedures in clinical pathology; just think of the number of PAP-smears that are performed each year. Yet, they have been difficult to capture digitally.

Relative to biopsies and resection pieces, cytology specimens are easy to obtain. Because of this, they would be a prime candidate to be prepared locally and digitized (by staff with limited, basic technical training). The specimens could subsequently be sent online to and screened at central treatment facilities where advanced analytical capabilities are available. Moreover, whereas biopsies result in a block of tissue that can usually still be accessed should something problematic occur with the original slide or slide(s), there is no such security with cytological specimens. If a cytology slide is lost or damaged in transit to the laboratory where it is to be viewed, the specimen must be collected again, if possible. The dearth of actual tissue collected is also an issue with respect to using cytology slides for educational purposes. Whereas a single block of tissue could potentially supply numerous glass slides to be used by a class of medical students, rarely does such a luxury exist for cytological specimens.

5.1 Diagnosis and Staging of Disease

These three reasons, among others, make cytology examinations one of the most obvious use cases for digital pathology. Unfortunately, there also are difficulties inherent in imaging cytological specimens, relative to biopsies. One relates to biopsy specimens typically being embedded in paraffin to generate a single uniform plane of tissue [6], whereas cytology specimens are inherently 3-dimensional due to cell clustering. This variability in specimen thickness causes problems with focussing, staining, and other image preparation steps. Another problem once again relates to the relatively small number of cells that typically are collected with a cytological specimen, such that cells will commonly be distributed widely across the slide or WSI. Whereas a trained, experienced pathologist should be able to identify which group of cells should be focussed upon, a digital scanner and the preprocessing steps that must be taken to prepare the virtual slide may not. As such, areas of prime interest might not be properly focussed, magnified, "stained," or otherwise prepped.

To date, little research has been done to validate the use of whole slide imaging for cytological specimens relative to traditional (glass slide) methods. Two studies comparing digital and glass slides have recently been published, both of them by the same research group. In the former, Bui et al. [7] had three pathologists and four cytotechnologists examine 11 cervicovaginal Papanicolaou (PAP) smears (Thin-Prep and SurePath) that were then scanned at ×20, ×40 and ×40 z-stack digital magnifications using a BioImagene iScan Coreo Au 3.0 scanner. The digital images then were viewed on a computer equipped with an Intel Pentium 3.44-GHz processor, with 1-GB RAM and 64-MB VRAM and a display monitor with 1,600 × 1,024 pixel resolution, and both the diagnosis and time to diagnosis recorded. These results were compared against manual reading of the same glass slides, at a later date, by the same observers (Fig. 5.1).

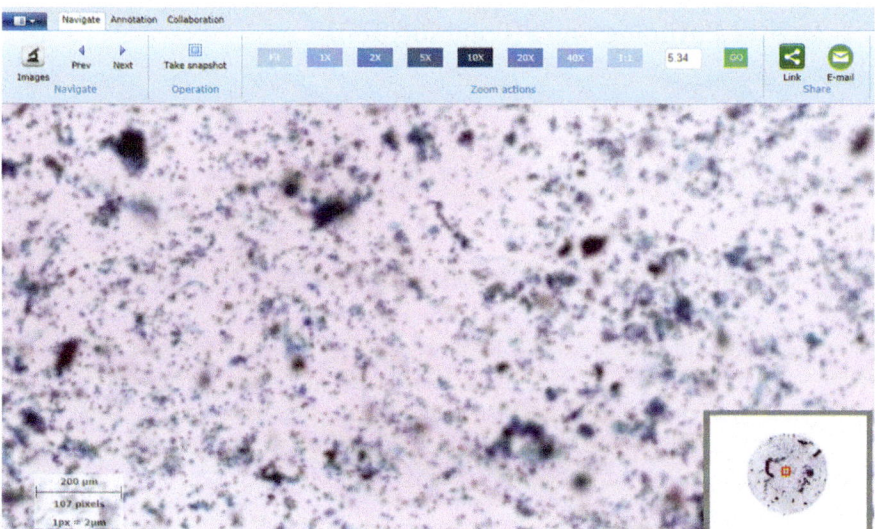

Fig. 5.1 A typical representation of a scanned cytology sample: some areas are in focus, some are not

In the second study, 22 de-identified previously screened and diagnosed cases were included, including both non-gynecological and gynecological slides [8]. Glass slides were digitalized using Aperio ScanScope XT (×20 and ×40). Three cytopathologists with and three without (3) digital experience, four cytotechnologists, and two senior pathology residents initially diagnosed the digital slides independently. Glass slides were read and recorded separately 1–3 days later. Once again, the accuracy of diagnosis and time to diagnosis were recorded. In both studies, glass slides out-performed WSI, and WSI took longer. For example, in the latter study, the diagnosis was accurate in 93 versus 86 % of cases, using glass versus digital slides. Though both techniques did well at recognizing positive cases (97.5 vs. 95.8 % for glass and digital slides, respectively), they did less well with negative cases (87.5 vs. 76.0 %, respectively), which is where the two approaches clearly differed. The average time required to read each slide also was roughly 1.5 min longer with WSI. However, the authors concluded from both studies that the problems with WSI were fixable, largely dependent upon increasing the speed of WSI capture and viewing, and generating better quality slides. They noted that only 10 % of the WSI were actually of poor quality [8] and did not comment on how many glass slides were not selected or had been tossed previously because they had been inadequate.

From these early results, what is clear is that, yes, considerable work still needs to be done to bring digital pathology to a level where it can be used with cytological specimens. On the other hand, the difference between where digital pathology is now and where it needs to be is not that great, so long as developers and investigators follow the same general validation guidelines recommended by the CAP for WSI use in standard pathology practice [8, 9].

5.2 Digital Pathology as a Teaching Tool

Chapter 3 discussed both the ease and effectiveness of using digital pathology as a teaching tool, as well as the numerous advantages. One professional school that has adopted it wholeheartedly is a school of podiatric medicine in New York.

5.2.1 New York College of Podiatric Medicine

Digital pathology, in the context of a 16-week course in basic mechanisms and systemic pathology, has now become one of the primary teaching tools at the New York College of Podiatric Medicine (NYCPM) [10]. The essential components of the digital pathology experience are (1) a laboratory in which core exercises are assigned for students to complete; (2) classroom access to computers for all students in small groups; (3) specialized software to access slides by virtual microscopy; (4) additional software that allows them to capture/download and edit slides for later presentation and sharing of observations; and (5) a course-specific (wiki) Web site (http://pathlab2014.wikifoundry.com) that allows them to enter and share their observations with every other student in the class outside of class time. For these purposes, the department's glass slide pathology collection was converted to the VM system (Olympus) for virtual viewing.

Laboratory sessions begin with a brief introduction to the essential features of the assigned digital slides, including slides demonstrating normal histology of each tissue. The students then work in groups of four, looking at the slides at their computer stations via virtual microscopy, as well as reviewing assigned references in *Wheater's Basic Pathology* and *Curran's Atlas of Histopathology*, with additional major atlases also available in the room (e.g., Sandritter and Damjanov). Toward the end of each session, new slides that demonstrate the same pathology but are not among the collection they already have viewed are projected onto the students' computer screens for open discussion across the entire class. For each slide, students are asked to volunteer their opinions about what they see, and what the likely pathology is and represents, from a disease perspective. Meanwhile, all other students are encouraged to agree or disagree with the initially expressed views and to explain why. The instructor guides the discussion with probing questions, as necessary—like "do you agree that this is subcutaneous tissue?" "do you agree that these are lymphocytes?" "do you agree that this is malignant change?" and always "why (do you agree or disagree)?" The discussion continues for each slide until a diagnostically accurate consensus is reached, aided by the instructor.

Advantages of this system are both numerous and undeniable. First, rather than four students taking brief turns examining glass slides, and perhaps not even visualizing the same field, using slides that differ from group to group, they are all able to visualize, on their computers, the same slide at the same time. Second, they can bring up images showing normal tissue and the assigned patient's pathology, side by side, to compare and contrast them, thereby more easily identifying the areas and characteristics of normal tissue and diseased tissue. Third, the students have access not only to slides in the NYCPM collection, but from collections housed at other universities, including collections at the Mt. Sinai School of Medicine, Albert Einstein College of Medicine, Ben Gurion University, and, via the course Web site (wiki), the University of Indiana and University of Iowa. Fourth, using programs like Paint, Image Manager, and Adobe, they have the capability to modify each slide—for example, to cut and paste significant areas, and to annotate, underline, circle, or add arrows; however, they wish to preserve their value-added versions of each slide. Fifth, via the online wiki Web site to which all students have 24/7 access, they can enter their personally modified slides and make them available to all, along with their comments and annotations. As such, all slides can be shared by all; modified and improved by all; downloaded and saved by all, either singly or as part of their own illustrated MS-Word notes or PowerPoint presentations; and, ultimately, studied by all.

5.2.2 Universal Education

Yet another advantage of a digital reference collection is that this digital educational tool can be used off-site, no matter the distance from the home university where it was created. All that is needed for those wishing to use it is to have computer access and have been allowed to register for the course Web site.

In the survey of the literature we conducted while writing this book, we found that education plays a role in virtually all digital pathology setups. Whether it is for sharing information with colleagues, or the formal offering of a course (as in the case of NYCPM), or in the training of pathology residents, or in continuing medical education for pathologists already in practice, it makes sense to use the infrastructure in place and get as much use out of it as possible.

Continuing medical education is an extremely important application, for a variety of reasons. For example, rare tumors are a fact of life, and in rural areas or small countries they may only appear once every so many years. They also might not be observed at all during a pathologist's formal years of training. It is useful, therefore, for practicing pathologists to be able to regularly update their skills by viewing pathology on their computer screen. The pathology can come from a patient who lives halfway around the world but who has a rare lesion of interest. Education then goes together with the construction of biobanks (see Chap. 3), whereby one can use the biobank as a study tool to stay current in diagnostic protocols.

This brings us back to telepathology, for which there also is an undeniable educational component. Initially, set up to assist in areas where pathology services are sparsely available, it stands to reason that the institute that is on the submitting end of the telepathology workflow uses the information it receives back, in terms of primary diagnoses and second opinions, to update its own knowledge base/skill set and pass it on to its associates and affiliates.

5.3 Telepathology in Developing Countries

One of the harsh social realities of life on Earth is that huge discrepancies exist in the standard of living and access to technical advances in different countries and regions. And in no field is this observed more than in the field of Medicine. For example, whereas almost 8,000 magnetic resonance image (MRI) scanners serve a US population of less than 320 million, in India, there are only about 600 units serving more than 1.2 billion people [11–13]. Per population, this translates to almost 26 MRI units per million in the US versus just 0.5 units per million in India, a more than 50-fold difference. Little can be done to alter such discrepancies in the availability of MRI units, which require that patients have physical access to the machine for it to be useful. This is not the case with DPUs, however, because slides are much more easily transported from place to place than people are; all a given region needs is a central DPU to create WSI from these slides; and, once made, these slides can be transmitted anywhere that has a computer to obtain specialist opinions, provided the necessary bandwidth requirements are fulfilled.

Two great examples of this at work are in Egypt and Haiti, the latter considered one of the poorest countries on Earth [14].

5.3.1 E-Education and Telepathology in Egypt

One interesting case of digital pathology being used in a developing country is a collaboration that has been established between Egypt and Italy [15]. The Egyptian partner is the IHC, an institute dating back to 1903. The project has been done in collaboration with the Egyptian Ministry of Health and the IHC. The concept of applying telemedicine programs at the IHC was born 12 years ago at a conference organized by the WHO in Cairo in Dec. 2001, with initial implementation taking place in 2003. The telemedicine project was actually divided into four phases, telepathology being the first (other areas include tele-echocardiography, teleradiology, and tele-endoscopy). Due to the success of the project, a new DPU was established in the faculty of medicine at Cairo University in 2009.

Dr. Ayad, director of the DPU, presented his experiences at the Pathology Visions 2013 conference in San Antonio, TX, USA. In the program, all teaching students' slides were scanned to create a Teaching Digital Pathology Library which was made available on the Web site of the Faculty of Medicine, Cairo University. The material within this Digital Pathology Library is to be used for:

(a) Routine learning in all histopathology classes
(b) e-learning by our undergraduate students, to be accessed either at home or in the new highly equipped Student Library (replacing the slide boxes formerly provided to students).

Routine scanning of all interesting cases (recent and archived) was done to create a huge Digital Pathology Library, which again was made available on the Web site of the Faculty of Medicine, Cairo University. The material of this Digital Pathology Library again is to be used for e-learning by our postgraduate students, divided into levels so as to be suitable for Masters degree and MD candidates. Moreover, a plan is in place to ultimately make this material accessible to postgraduate students outside our University, as well.

Another application of scanned slides that has already changed is the method of teaching pathology classes, so that slides can be accessed virtually via computers by either under- or post-graduate students. Even the professors have become more acquainted with this new technology involving digital files rather than ordinary microscope slides.

While establishing the Digital Pathology Library in the Faculty of Medicine at Cairo University, difficulties concerning the quality of the slides produced for routine pathological examination became apparent. In particular, the scanner has been able to detect numerous minute technical errors that could not be detected during routine analog microscopic examination. This, in turn, has led to a call for dramatic improvements in slide quality, demonstrating how the use of virtual pathology has enhanced routine examination practices as well.

With respect to telepathology for quality assurance (QA) and second opinions (expert-to-expert consultations), provisional agreements have also been made with several, different highly specialized pathology centers in developing countries (like Italy, the UK, and the USA) to consult on our cases. The IHC is now trying to increase the number of centers of expertise that will cooperate with it. Many centers have been quite eager to participate, once they understand what the system is and how it works.

In the Department of Pathology at the IHC, the number of cases examined annually exceeds 1,500 (roughly five cases daily). Among these, one case per week requires a higher level of external consultation, involving highly specialized consultants. Consequently, the expected number of difficult cases presenting to the Department of Pathology at IHC is approximately 50 annually.

The average cost of sending physical slides to just one American or European center is approximately US$100 each. Adding this transportation fee to the average fee for a consultation (approximately US$150) yields a total consultation cost estimate, just to handle the typical 50 cases per year, of roughly US$12.500 annually. Moreover, this number is likely a gross underestimate. Given that such challenging cases are usually sent to two or three centers to garner more opinions, this figure would likely be multiplied two to three times, up to almost US$40,000 annually. In fact, the exact costs were approximately US$187,500 over the five-year duration of the project, compared to the extremely low cost (US$5,000) of establishing the entire telepathology unit.

Finally, another channel of telepathology that the team in Cairo is establishing is offering second opinions (expert-to-expert consultations). The aim is to create agreements with different pathology centers in different surrounding Arabic countries that have only a limited number of specialized pathologists (like Palestine, Sudan, Yemen and Libya) to consult on their cases. In this way, IHC may fill the role of a pivot center between these countries and more-advanced western countries. Despite the recent unstable political status developments in Egypt, the progress in implementation and expansion of our digital pathology project is very promising.

5.3.2 Heavy Lifting in Port-au-Prince, Haiti

What if all patients could have an accurate, timely, and informative diagnosis of their disease, regardless of their circumstances or home? While the US FDA currently prohibits the use of digital pathology for primary diagnosis in the US, it still offers the possibility for US-based laboratories to apply digital pathology in their workflow when it concerns tissues not collected from US-based patients. This is exactly what people in Seattle have done in collaboration with healthcare organizations in Haiti.

Gregory S. Henderson, MD, Ph.D., is the founder and president of PathForceDx in Seattle, WA. He is passionate about digital pathology because of the unique combination of technology, image analysis, and potential for sharing. He observed that, while slide scanners and digitally imaged slides have existed for at least 10 years (and computerized anatomic pathology reporting systems for almost 40 years), the real challenge in poor areas around the world (those that possibly stand to benefit the most) is to make these new technologies easy to use and readily accessible.

A solution was created using Simagis Slide Image Viewer and Storage, the PathCentral Cloud Based Information System, as well as a team of freelancing and volunteer pathologists. Since June 2012, using the Power of the PathForceDx Solutions and Network, over 700 female patients in Haiti have received lifesaving diagnoses from pathologists in the US and Canada who never left their own offices.

It must be said that, at this point, tissue samples are still sent to the continental US for processing, scanning, and (virtual) distribution. In order to truly scale this concept, it should be possible to develop a low-priced, robust, and easy-to-use slide scanner that can be deployed in local areas, to be operated by RNs or EMTs with only basic training, rather than highly qualified laboratory technicians and engineers. Indeed, such a device would be extremely useful for both military and civilian (e.g., disaster relief) applications alike.

This being said, networks have been established within other countries as well, including China [16], providing pathology consultation services across much of the country; and Kenya, providing services to several other countries in Africa [17]. Adding another exciting dimension to this is the potential to train physicians in developing countries.

5.4 Quality Control and Assurance

Quality issues are amplified in digital pathology. This provides an opportunity for robust quality metrics to be put in place to facilitate continuous improvement. An important part of preprocessing is identifying and removing artefacts created by tissue sampling, processing and staining. Artefacts are glass slide scratches, dust particles, hairs, ink, and air bubbles, but also the glass slide edge, the slide label, etc. Digital pathology could be a particularly useful tool to identify and study artifacts, from a quality control perspective. Techniques and algorithms could be designed specifically in this way to detect artifacts, categorize them, and even separate staining signals from artifacts [18]. This could lead to better strategies to cope with artifacts in general—a fact of life in pathology, and not always avoidable in the heat of the surgical battlefield.

There is a significant gap between what has been demonstrated to be best practices in anatomic pathology and what is typically observed in common practice, with respect to the accuracy and reliability of diagnoses. Current QA programs may have topped out in their ability to close this gap significantly. External peer reviews by specialists can set a new standard of quality, in that they will allow common practices at one site or in one department to be evaluated by others. However, this practice is not currently being performed to any significant extent, largely because of the difficulties and costs associated with transporting slides and/or specialists. Using whole slide digital imaging as an enabling technology can provide a confidential, cost-effective, user-friendly means to perform external peer reviews by specialists and help to close this gap.

Intra-institutional clinical peer reviews are a primary QA process that physicians use to review their performance. Studies have shown that peer-review programs and related organizational factors explain up to 18 % of the variation in standardized measures for quality and patient safety. A well-designed external peer-review program can demonstrate that a self-regulatory process is an effective means to promote quality and patient safety [19]. Digital pathology can help to improve QA in pathology applications. For example, using digital pathology and QA Case Review Software with QualityStar™ external QA program, it is now possible to

- Randomly select (1–10 % of cases) and digitize slides from retrospectively de-identified cases for external peer review for QA
- Assemble, de-identify, and upload cases to an encrypted Dell data server for review by QualityStar™ AP specialists at pre-qualified academic medical centers; and
- Have AP specialists capture key metrics using the ADASP Recommendation for QA and Improvement in Surgical and Autopsy Pathology guidelines.

Reviews are collected, metrics are converted, and the mean and ± two standard deviations (SD) are calculated. Results are reported monthly in multiple graphic formats. Digital pathology, therefore, is an easy way to perform QA assessments within individual departments, identify departments and areas within departments wherein diagnoses are less accurate, and ultimately enhance the diagnostic process and optimize patient management at the outset, rather than later when time has been lost and costs accumulated.

5.5 Tremendous Potential

It is said that there are two types of pathologist: those who feel that digital pathology is the future and are willing to start working with it today; and those who feel that digital pathology is the future, but that it will always remain so. As can be seen from the examples in this chapter, more and more practitioners are starting to fall into the former of these two camps.

What never ceases to amaze those of us in the field is the chameleon-like properties of digital pathology, capable of adapting to almost any setting and any use. Whether it is in medically advanced metropolitan centers like New York, or poverty-struck developing countries like Haiti; whether it is used for education, primary diagnosis, biomarker identification, second opinions, QA, or research; and whether it is used for surgical, biopsy or cytology specimens, there is a case to be made for digital pathology, and those who adopt its use appear to benefit because of it.

Chapter 6, the final chapter, describes how monumental that impact could be and introduces even more ways in which digital pathology will one day, soon, leave its mark.

References

1. Chemotherapy: Response and Survival Data, 2nd ed. Medical College of Wisconsin (2014)
2. Wang, X.Y., Zuo, D., Sarkar, D., Fisher, P.B.: Blockade of cytotoxic T-lymphocyte antigen-4 as a new therapeutic approach for advanced melanoma. Expert Opin. Pharmacother. **12**, 2695–2706 (2011)
3. Balch, C., Montgomery, J.S., Paik, H.I., et al.: New anti-cancer strategies: epigenetic therapies and biomarkers. Front Biosci. **10**, 1897–1931 (2005)
4. Amado, R.G., Wolf, M., Peeters, M., et al.: Wild-type KRAS is required for panitumumab efficacy in patients with metastatic colorectal cancer. J. Clin. Oncol. **26**, 1626–1634 (2008)
5. Galluzzi, L., Senovilla, L., Zitvogel, L., Kroemer, G.: The secret ally: immunostimulation by anticancer drugs. Nat. Rev. Drug Discov. **11**, 215–233 (2012)
6. Thrall, M., Pantanowicz, L., Khalbuss, W.: Telecytology: clinical applications, current challenges, and future benefits. J. Pathol. Inform. **2**, 51. Epub 2011 Dec 26 (2011). doi:10.4103/2153-3539.91129
7. Bui, M.M., Stephenson, C.L.: What is new in the evaluation of diagnostic digital cytopathology in cervicovaginal smears? J. Pathol. Inform. **4**, 18 (2013)
8. House, J.C., Henderson-Jackson, E.B., Johnson, J.O., et al.: Diagnostic digital cytopathology: are we ready yet? J. Pathol. Inform. **4**, 28 (2013)
9. Pantanowicz, L., Sinard, J.H., Henricks, W.H., et al.: Validating whole slide imaging for diagnostic purposes in pathology: guideline from the College of American Pathologists Pathology and Laboratory Quality Center. Arch. Pathol. Lab. Med. **137**, 1710–1722 (2013)
10. Leifer, Z.: The use of virtual microscopy, slide modification and a wiki in pathology education (2014)
11. Number of Magnetic Resonance Imaging (MRI) units and Computed Tomography (CT) scanners: selected countries, selected years 1990–2009. Centers for Disease Control and Prevention (2014)
12. Jankharia, G.R.: Commentary—radiology in India: the next decade. Indian J. Radiol. Imaging **18**, 189–191 (2008)
13. List of countries by population. Wikipedia (2014)
14. GDP per capita, PPP (current international $), World Development Indicators database, World Bank. The World Bank. 8-5-2014. Accessed 29 May 2014
15. Ayad, E., Sicurello, F.: Telepathology in emerging countries pilot project between Italy and Egypt. Diagn. Pathol. **3**, S2 (2008)
16. Digital Pathology in China. Digital Pathology Association (2014)
17. Dimaras, H., Dimba, E.A.O., Waweru, W., Githanga, J., Kimani, K.: Digital cancer pathology in Africa. Lancet. Oncolog. **14**, e289–e290 (2013)
18. Kothari, S., Phan, J.H., Wang, M.D.: Eliminating tissue-fold artifacts in histopathological whole-slide images for improved image-based prediction of cancer grade. J. Pathol. Inform. **4**, 22 (2013)
19. Edwards, M.T.: The objective impact of clinical peer review on hospital quality and safety. Am. J. Med. Qual. **26**, 110–119 (2011)

Chapter 6
A Bright Future

Abstract Digital pathology is an idea whose time has come. The hardware keeps getting better year after year, and enough companies now have invested in this new field to gather the critical mass necessary to turn digital pathology into a mainstream technique. But this is not enough. What remains is for digital pathology to significantly impact the way medical diagnoses are made and patients managed on a large scale.

Keywords Digital pathology · Medical systems biology · 3D imaging · Micro-CT · Spectral imaging · Digital pathology future · Digital pathology applications

6.1 The 5 %/$2.4 Billion Challenge

At the 2013 Digital Pathology Association's meeting in San Antonio, Texas, in an inspiring keynote presentation, Mark Priebe discussed the concept of a "5 %/$2.4 billion challenge." The 5 % refers to the number of cases of misdiagnosis to be averted, and the $2.4 billion the cost savings such an accomplishment could achieve.

More specifically, because roughly 1.6 million pathology cases are reviewed every year in the USA, the 5 % translates into 80,000 cases. This 5 % is a conservative estimate of the percentage of pathology cases for which a major misdiagnosis occurs upon first review.

It is well known that many cases exist in which a diagnosis made in one pathology department is not corroborated by another. Swapp et al. [1] in their review of almost 72,000 (71,811) cases assessed at two centers found that there was a *major* disagreement in the diagnosis in 457 cases, resulting in some change in the management approach, representing 0.6 % of the total. Other estimates of major disagreement have been higher to much higher. In fact, across a host of other studies conducted over the past two decades, estimates of major discrepancies with second opinions have ranged from 1.3 % to as high as 30 %, averaging roughly

10 %. Such changes in diagnosis or disease-stage estimations have not only clinical, but societal cost implications, especially when there is some time lag between the first and second pathology assessments. For example, with cancers, the cost of a change in diagnosis increases as the stage of tumor increases, and the average cost of any change in diagnosis is $30,000 [2, 3]. That $30,000 per case, multiplied by 80,000 cases (conservatively reducing the 10 % mean estimate of major discrepancies with second opinions to 5 % of all cases), accounts for $2.4 billion wasted healthcare expenses, hence Priebe's 5 %/$2.4 billion challenge.

Five percent—or 80,000 US cases per year representing 2.4 B US dollars in wasted healthcare costs—is a large enough gap to warrant our attention. Note that production = cases = patients = people. The goal is to close the significant gap that currently exists between best demonstrated practices and common practice in the accuracy of diagnoses within anatomic pathology. Enabling technologies like WSI provides a confidential, cost-effective, user-friendly means by which to facilitate external peer reviews and help close this gap.

6.2 New Frontiers

As stated earlier, as far as digital pathology has come over the past 10–15 years, and as many new inroads, it has made, what we have seen so far is, almost certainly, just scratching the surface. Just like photocopiers have recently been developed that not only copy 3-dimensional hard structures, like functional tools, but "print" them half a world away or potentially at an off-world space station [4], something most could not even have envisioned a few years ago, there are so many areas in which digital pathology may revolutionize the practice of medicine and beyond. Below is a brief look at some ground-breaking areas and fields in which digital pathology has already taken a prominent role.

6.2.1 Medical Systems Biology

The emergence of digital whole slide imaging and analysis is not the only way in which the fields of histopathology and pathology are changing. Another area in which digital pathology, including digital imaging and analysis, is demonstrating increasing value is in the very new but rapidly emerging field of *medical systems biology*. Largely since the year 2000, systems biology has emerged an inter-disciplinary field of study that focuses on complex interactions within biological systems, using a holistic approach to biological and biomedical research. One of the primary objectives of systems biology is to model and discover how cells, tissues, and organisms function as a system, including the workings of metabolic and cell signaling networks [5], rather than studying them at a given fixed moment in time, as is traditional under a standard microscope. It then makes heavy use of mathematical and computational models to generate a better and more systematic understanding of the interactions between various bodily systems.

One recent example of how digital pathology has facilitated this process has been using 3-dimensional tissue cultures, combined with semiautomated standardized histology and automatic slide imaging and analysis to study wound healing. To accomplish this, in their study of re-epithelialization following a punch biopsy, Safferling et al. [6] created a technical analysis pipeline of 3-dimensional organotypic wound models, standardized immunohistology, fluorescent whole slide imaging, image analysis, multiplex protein analytics, and computational systems biological modeling. Ninety-two 3D full-thickness skin-wound models, consisting of keratinocytes and fibroblasts, were tracked in time via two-step time-lag fluorescence staining. This allowed the investigators to visualize epidermal wound-healing spatiotemporally and in three dimensions, specifically assessing cell proliferation, migration, and differentiation, so as to derive a consistent theory about how these three processes are intertwined.

6.2.2 Three-Dimensional WSI

Three-dimensional whole slide imaging is another rapidly emerging field of pathology. As a gross over-simplification, 3D imaging is accomplished by stacking multiple focus planes. Advantages over traditionally paraffin-embedded 3D sections are numerous, but include being much simpler and less time-consuming. Advantages of 3D over 2D imaging are that it allows for better delineation of the spatial distributions and structural interactions of various tissue elements [7]. WSI technologies and rendering software have now improved to the point that 3D reconstruction of large structures at a microscopic scale from hundreds of serial sections is now possible. However, there are numerous challenges to this, which include dealing with section registration, tissue quality, the effects of tissue processing and sectioning, and the huge amount of data that can be generated [8]. However, processing complex tissues and managing huge datasets is something that pioneers in the digital pathology field have been improving at steadily. And the potential benefits of 3D digital imaging, in terms of understanding and classifying disease, are too great to be ignored.

In one just-published study, for example, Onozato et al. [9] attempted to better define histological subtypes of lung adenocarcinoma by studying four formalin-fixed human lung cancer resections. After paraffin-embedded tissues were sectioned using a Kurabo-Automated tissue sectioning machine, serial sections were automatically stained and scanned with a whole slide imaging system. The resulting image stacks were 3D-reconstructed using Pannoramic Viewer software (http://www.3dhistech.com). On inspection, the investigators found that two of the four specimens contained islands of tumor cells detached in alveolar spaces, a finding that had not been described in any preexisting adenocarcinoma classifications. Moreover, these tumor cell islands extended deep into the tissue, interconnected with each other and with the main tumor via a solid pattern that was surrounded by the islands. These findings caused the investigators to question whether the islands of tumor cells should be classified into a solid pattern within the current classification scheme, a change that could have prognostic implications [10].

In another example of the benefits of 3D over 2D WSI, it may be that certain low-power morphologic features that help distinguish benign from malignant follicular lymphoid proliferations may be enhanced by 3D analysis [8]. Three-dimensional reconstructions from WSIs also would facilitate estimates of coronary vessel narrowing, since 2D sections do not indicate the angle of the vessel relative to the section plane [8].

6.2.3 Spectral Imaging

What spectral imaging can offer over conventional methods is improved detection, validation, separation, and quantitation [11]. For example, a researcher can record the spectrum of auto-fluorescence and the spectrum of his desired signal or stain. With this spectral information, an image can be separated to reveal any auto-fluorescence, and false-positives can be prevented.

Spectral imaging can be divided into multispectral imaging, hyper-spectral imaging, and ultra-spectral imaging, according to its spectral resolution, and the number, width, and contiguousness of bands [12]. This technique can acquire reflectance, absorption, or fluorescence spectra for each pixel in the image, which can be used to detect biological and pathological changes in tissues that cannot be identified with traditional gray- or color-imaging methods [12].

A spectral imaging system has four main parts: collection optics or instruments; a spectral dispersion element; a detector; and a system control and data collection module [12]. The spectral dispersion element (a spectrometer, a filter, or an interferometer) is the heart of the system that enables separation of the light into different wavelengths [12]. A real slide scanner does not exist today, but various microscopic multispectral or hyper-spectral systems have been developed; for example, the HSi-300/HSi440C hyper-spectral imaging systems of Gooch and Housego, the Prism and Reflector Imaging Spectroscopy System (PARISS) hyper-spectral imaging system of LightForm, and the Nuance/Vectra multiplexing microscopes of Perkin Elmer. For a detailed comparison of the different available spectral systems, the review published by Li et al. [12] is a great start.

Regardless of the hardware technology used, a spectral imager delivers image sets (x, y, and wavelength intensity) that contain spectral information at every pixel [11]. While spectra containing hundreds or even thousands of spectrally distinct intensities at each pixel can be acquired, such imaging is generally of less practical use than it might seem [11]. Capturing a subset of the available spectral information is usually sufficient [11].

Spectral imaging opens up a whole new array of possibilities, such as digital simulation of staining [13], the coupling of spectral imaging with fluorescence and white-light microscopy [14], and the development of new approaches to antibody conjugation [15].

6.2.4 Extending the Pathology Value Chain, Upstream, and Downstream

Histopathology plays a major part in the correct clinical diagnosis of a large number of diseases, among which cancer accounts for a large percentage. The diagnosis that is rendered typically determines not only what further treatment the patient is offered, but how that treatment is framed (e.g., as potentially curative versus life-prolonging versus palliative) because of how the pathological appearance of the tumor predicts patient survival. The histopathological assessment of tissue is therefore a critical node in the medical treatment path. There is also a real potential for the pathological diagnosis to extend beyond the clinical setting into research, especially as researchers and clinicians strive to find more effective anticancer treatments.

Cancer classification is usually made based upon the morphological and histopathological appearance of the tumor, taking into account parameters like tumor size and heterogeneity. A large drawback of traditional histopathology is its relatively high level of inter-observer variability. Lack of objective data results in arbitrary acceptance of one set of criteria over another, whenever there is no inter-institutional or consensus gold standard [16, 17]. In practice, one senior experienced pathologist at an individual institution usually serves as the final authority. It is then a big challenge to reduce diagnostic variability with conventional interpretative techniques. More objective methods could lead to a resolution of this problem. One such method is mass spectroscopy imaging (commonly called mass spec. imaging or MSI).

MSI is a relatively new molecular imaging technology that enables the direct analysis of the spatial distribution of hundreds of molecules in a tissue section. It has been used successfully to study pathology, fundamental biological processes, and pharmacology at the tissue level in both animals and humans [18–24]. During MSI analysis, the tissue section is overlaid with a virtual grid, and at every grid point, a mass spectrum is acquired directly from the underlying tissue.

Tools used in digital pathology can help to facilitate the integration of novel techniques like MSI in daily clinical applications. Through digital pathology platforms, all the elements necessary for MSI to be adopted by a routine pathology laboratory can be entered into the standardized workflow.

Digital pathology can assist with MSI profiling right from the start: guiding an MSI-instrument toward a limited number of interesting pixels can be done via on-slide annotations. The selected areas can then be converted into device-specific configuration files for the MSI hardware to use to determine scanning areas. Profiled areas are then based upon site-specific histology. In addition, this can significantly reduce any reluctance typically associated with new technology. Digital pathology also helps to reduce the costs of MSI, because it limits the number of pixels that need to be measured (the laser is not as heavily used), resulting in increased speed.

Once a sufficient sample size has been analyzed with MSI, a library of profiles can be constructed. These profiles need to be validated. The logical course of action is to involve the pathologist again, to do a blinded study to see whether observations by the pathologist match the predicted analysis of the MSI screening algorithm. However, in order to capture the pathologist's input, it is best to deploy digital pathology techniques as well. In this way, side-by-side (MSI pathology) observations can be compared off-line in an unbiased manner. It also allows for easy inter- and intra-observer reproducibility studies.

Much has been written about the integration of next-generation sequencing (NGS) into traditional pathology practices [25, 26]. We believe, however, that MSI could offer an even more exciting information layer to complement the pathologist's view. There are two reasons for this. First, MSI does not destroy tissue features; locational information is kept intact, and the position of features relative to each other may very well play a role in disease outcomes. Second, MSI does not target nucleic acids; and, as such, it casts a wider net. Stroma and inter-cellular features have now been recognized to play a role in tumor pathology as well [27]. However, by definition, next-generation sequencing can only capture features that can be sequenced.

6.3 Hope for the Third World

Imagine saving a life half a world away just by turning on your computer.

As stated in Chap. 5, digital pathology is now being used to help healthcare specialists in industrialized countries to provide expert medical opinions to those in developing countries, where there is often a profound lack of physicians of any kind, let alone specialists. For example, thanks to PathForceDx in Seattle, Washington, since June 2012, over 700 female patients in Haiti have received life-saving diagnoses from pathologists in the USA and Canada who never left their own offices. This all was accomplished using the PathForceDx Solutions and Network, along with a Simagis Slide Image Viewer. Similarly, via a collaboration between Italy and Egypt via the Italian Hospital in Cairo, expert pathologist opinions are now being provided for patients not only in Egypt, but in other African countries as well [28]. Similar collaborative networks are now up and running in Nairobi [29] and China [30].

This is, of course, just the tip of the iceberg. As digital pathology systems become more mainstream, and pathologists more accustomed to them, such services could be provided to developing countries worldwide. Think, for example, how such a network could be of help during infectious epidemics, allowing for the earlier detection of unusual pathogens via expert pathological reviews from multiple experts simultaneously. And think how such a system also could aid in the training of healthcare providers in poorer countries that lack the facilities to provide such training themselves.

6.4 Digital Pathology DIY

We hope this book has helped to convince you that digital pathology is the wave of the future. For those willing to dive in, we can now formulate a preliminary road map about how to best prepare your own digital pathology workflow. We offer these suggestions based upon our own experiences and the experiences of others.

In general, you should start with the most experienced users within your organization. Conversely, you should limit yourself to a limited number of very specific use cases and specimen types in the beginning (GU, endocrine, liver, head and neck, etc.).

Once users become familiar with this first phase, upscaling can take place. At this point, you should involve more users (or better, let the initial collaborators spread the word and have new participants come to you), and expand to more disease and specimen types. You should attempt to scan all cases for these groups, so as to prevent parallel workflows.

Review and validate the digital slides, but make sure to request glass slides whenever you feel this is still required or prudent. See if the usage of glass slides for diagnostic purposes decreases over time. The most likely evolution is that a (preferably low) plateau will be reached. Make sure to record and evaluate performance data. Once you are satisfied with operations, approach more sites and groups and repeat the process.

This may be too simple an explanation. Clearly, there is more involved: hardware must be evaluated and purchased (no single vendor exists today that can satisfy all needs), funds must be found, physical space must be allocated for new equipment, etc. Yet all of these are straightforward steps within a normal procurement cycle, and not that different from the purchase of a new auto-cleaver or a microtome.

Probably, the most important thing to realize is that digital pathology does not happen overnight. You cannot pull a switch one day and transport your department into the digital pathology age the next. It is therefore crucial that other peripheral factors are handled properly. Make sure that you have bar-coding in place before you switch from your optical microscopes. Plan your new workflow (it will be different once you go digital). Talk with your LIS-vendor about integrating your digital pathology solution into their service modules. Do not forget to negotiate a solid maintenance contract with your digital pathology provider either; this is new technology that still has some kinks to be worked out. Some questions to ask:

- Do you qualify for free upgrades?
- Do they have a support hotline?
- Who performs validation assessments of the equipment once it is delivered?

Finally, talk to others. This book is filled with references from people who have travelled down this road already. It was our experience that most were very willing to assist us when we asked for help. Attending conferences may help as well, to familiarize yourself with the latest best practices. At the end of this book, we also have a brief list of digital pathology organizations that may assist you in your journey. Most have a (bi-annual) meeting. You may even run into one of the authors of this book there.

6.5 Final Conclusions

Digital pathology has experienced exponential growth, in terms of its technology and applications, since its inception just over a decade ago. Though it has yet to be approved for primary diagnostics, its values as a teaching tool, facilitator of second opinions and quality assurance reviews, and research are becoming, if not already, undeniable. It also offers the hope of providing pathology consultant and educational services to under-served areas, including regions of the world that could not possibly sustain this level of services otherwise.

And this is just the beginning, as its adoption by the also rapidly emerging fields of medical systems biology and 3D tissue imaging indicate.

We have shown how digital pathology not only has the potential to dramatically impact medical education and the delivery of health care, but also to exert an immensely positive influence worldwide, including countries and regions that normally fail to benefit from such technological advances.

Challenges exist, however, starting with convincing more pathologists about the added value and efficiency of this approach over traditional microscopic examinations, and standardization of the numerous techniques and technologies being developed.

Will digital pathology totally replace the standard microscope? Just like paper will remain, despite the overwhelming emergence of electronic readers in all their forms, microscopes and glass slides will probably have a place for years if not decades to come. However, it is clear that, with its countless advantages and tremendous flexibility, the use of and applications for digital pathology are sure to increase. The prospects are indeed exciting.

6.6 Learn More About Digital Pathology

There are a number of dedicated digital pathology resources around the Web, useful for learning more. Here are a few good sites for you to explore:

http://www.jpathinformatics.org/—Journal of Pathology Informatics
https://digitalpathologyassociation.org/—Digital Pathology Association
http://www.pathologyinformatics.com/—Association for Pathology Informatics

http://d-pathology.partners.org/iadp/index.htm—International Academy on Digital Pathology

http://www.wsi-conference.com—European Conference on Whole Slide Imaging

http://www.digitalpathology2014.org/—European Congress on Digital Pathology

http://www.openmicroscopy.org—An open source initiative to come up with a universal file format (OME TIFF) for whole slide imaging

http://www.openslide.org—An open source library to read any proprietary brightfield file format

http://en.wikipedia.org/wiki/Digital_pathology—An online continuously updated resource, with many extra references

References

1. Swapp, R.E., Aubry, M.C., Salomao, D.R., Cheville, J.C.: Outside case review of surgical pathology for referred patients: the impact on patient care. Arch. Pathol. Lab. Med. **137**, 233–240 (2013)
2. Elkin, E.: The cost of cancer care: how much do we spend and how can we spend it better? In: 34th Annual CTRC-AACR San Antonio Breast Cancer Symposium (2011)
3. Hassett, M.: Health care reform and cost control: practical and ethical considerations for cancer care providers. In: 34th Annual CTRC-AACR San Antonio Breast Cancer Symposium (2011)
4. Excell, J., Nathan, S.: The rise of additive manufacturing. The Engineer (2010). The original article is at http://www.theengineer.co.uk/in-depth/the-big-story/the-rise-of-additive-manufacturing/1002560.article
5. Bu, Z., Callaway, D.J.: Proteins move! Protein dynamics and long-range allostery in cell signaling. Adv. Protein Chem. Struct. Biol. **83**, 163–221 (2011)
6. Safferling, K., Sutterlin, T., Westphal, K., et al.: Wound healing revised: a novel reepithelialization mechanism revealed by in vitro and in silico models. J. Cell. Biol. **203**, 691–709 (2013)
7. Song, Y., Treanor, D., Bulpitt, A.J., Magee, D.R.: 3D reconstruction of multiple stained histology images. J. Pathol. Inform. **4**, S7 (2014)
8. Yagi, Y.: Challenges in whole slide image based 3D imaging (2014). http://tigacenter.bioquant.uni-heidelberg.de/tl_files/tigacenter/workshops/conference2013/Slides/Yukako%20Yagi%20%28MGH%29.pdf
9. Onozato, M.L., Klepeis, V.E., Yagi, Y., Mino-Kenudson, M.: A role of three-dimensional (3D)-reconstruction in the classification of lung adenocarcinoma. Anal. Cell. Pathol. (Amst) **35**, 79–84 (2012)
10. Onozato, M.L., Kovach, A.E., Yeap, B.Y., et al.: Tumor islands in resected early-stage lung adenocarcinomas are associated with unique clinicopathologic and molecular characteristics and worse prognosis. Am. J. Surg. Pathol. **37**, 287–294 (2013)
11. Levenson, R., Beechem, J., McNamara, G.: Spectral imaging in preclinical research and clinical pathology. Anal. Cell. Pathol. (Amsterdam) **35**, 339–361 (2012)
12. Li, Q., He.X., Wang, Y.: Review of spectral imaging technology in biomedical engineering: achievements and challenges. J Biomed. Opt. **18** (2013)
13. Bautista, P., Yagi, Y.: Digital simulation of staining in histopathology multispectral images: enhancement and linear transformation of spectral transmittance. J Biomed. Opt. **17** (2012)
14. Dolloff, N.G., Ma, X., Dicker, D.T.: Spectral imaging-based methods for quantifying autophagy and apoptosis. Canc. Biol. Therap. **12**, 349–356 (2011)
15. Guo, J., Wang, S., Dai, N., Teo, Y.N., Kool, E.T.: Multispectral labeling of antibodies with polyfluorophores on a DNA backbone and application in cellular imaging. Proc. Nat. Acad. Sci. U.S.A. **108**(9), 3493–3498 (2011)

16. Mahon, C., Brachtel, E., Cosatto, E., et al.: Mitotic figure recognition: agreement among pathologists and computerized detector. Anal. Cell. Pathol. (Amst) **35**, 97–100 (2012)
17. Raab, S.S., Meier, F.A., Zarbo, R.J., et al.: The "Big Dog" effect: variability assessing the causes of error in diagnoses of patients with lung cancer. J. Clin. Oncol. **24**, 2808–2814 (2006)
18. Shariatgorji, M., Svenningsson, P., Anderin, P.E.: Mass spectrometry imaging, an emerging technology in neuropsychopharmacology. Neuropsychopharmacology **39**, 34–49 (2014)
19. Sun, N., Walch, A.: Qualitative and quantitative mass spectrometry imaging of drugs and metabolites in tissue at therapeutic levels. Histochem. Cell. Biol. **140**, 93–104 (2013)
20. Nimesh, S., Mohattalage, S., Vincent, R., Kumarathasan, P.: Current status and future perspectives of mass spectrometry imaging. Int. J. Mol. Sci. **14**, 11277–11301 (2013)
21. Weaver, E.M., Hummon, A.B.: Imaging mass spectrometry: from tissue sections to cell cultures. Adv. Drug Deliv. Rev. **65**, 1039–1055 (2013)
22. Liu, J., Ouyang, Z.: Mass spectrometry imaging for biomedical applications. Anal. Bioanal. Chem. **405**, 5645–5653 (2013)
23. Norris, J.L., Caprioli, R.M.: Imaging mass spectrometry: a new tool for pathology in a molecular age. Proteomics Clin. Appl. **7**, 733–738 (2013)
24. Schwamborn, K., Caprioli, R.M.: Molecular imaging by mass spectrometry—looking beyond classical histology. Nat. Rev. Cancer **10**, 639–646 (2010)
25. Meldrum, C., Doyle, M.A., Tothill, R.W.: Next-generation sequencing for cancer diagnostics: a practical perspective. Clin. Biochem. Rev. **32**, 177–195 (2011)
26. Salto-Tellez, M., de Castro, D.G.: Next generation sequencing: a change of paradigm in molecular diagnostic validation. J. Pathol. (2014). doi: 10. 1002/path. 4365 [Epub ahead of print]
27. Gujam, F.J., Edwards, J., Mohammed, Z.M., Going, J.J., McMillan, D.C.: The relationship between the tumour stroma percentage, clinicopathological characteristics and outcome in patients with operable ductal breast cancer. Br. J. Cancer. **279**. doi: 10. 1038/bjc [Epub ahead of print]
28. Ayad, E., Sicurello, F.: Telepathology in emerging countries pilot project between Italy and Egypt. Diagn. Pathol. **3**, S2 (2008)
29. Dimaras, H., Dimba, E.A.O., Waweru, W., Githanga, J., Kimani, K.: Digital cancer pathology in Africa. Lancet Oncolog. **14**, e289–e290 (2013)
30. Digital Pathology in China. Digital Pathology Association (2014)

Retraction Note: Hardware and Software

Erratum to:
Chapter 2 in: Y. Sucaet and W. Waelput, *Digital Pathology,*
SpringerBriefs in Computer Science,
DOI 10.1007/978-3-319-08780-1_2

The authors have retracted this chapter published in Digital Pathology (Pages 15–29, DOI 10.1007/978-3-319-08780-1_2), as it contains multiple portions of text that have been duplicated from the OpenSlide website, http://openslide.org/. In particular, Sections 2.4.1.3, 2.4.1.4, 2.4.1.6 and 2.4.2.1 contain text that has been copied from the pages http://openslide.org/formats/leica/, http://openslide.org/formats/aperio/, http://openslide.org/formats/hamamatsu/ and http://openslide.org/formats/mirax/, without sufficient permission or attribution.

The whole chapter 'Hardware and Software' by Y. Sucaet and W. Waelput in Digital Pathology (2014), (pp. 15–29) is retracted and replaced by a new chapter based on author's request.

The online version of the original chapter can be found under
DOI 10.1007/978-3-319-08780-1_2

Chapter 2
Hardware and Software

Abstract Lest those interested in exploring the field not understand the nuts and bolts of the system, no book on digital technology is complete without some background on the available hardware and software. The field is changing rapidly and specific examples may be already obsolete at the time this book goes to press. At the same time, we have found that certain principles have remained constant for a relatively long time now, and we believe that providing readers with some general technical background will help on the path to implementing successful digital pathology solutions.

Keywords Digital pathology • Slide scanner • Tile scanner • Line scanner • File format • Medical imaging • WSI • DP • MRXS • NDPI • SVS • BIF

This chapter talks about the technology that is used to arrive at digital pathology. As the pathologist is dependent upon his microscope, so is the digital pathologist dependent upon a digital camera or slide scanner for the creation of a single, high-magnification digital image of an entire microscopic slide or whole slide image (WSI).

This chapter is split into two parts. In Sect. 2.1, we elaborate on the various hardware components necessary to acquire virtual slides. In Sect. 2.2, we survey the various approaches to data storage and file format organization that different vendors have developed.

2.1 How Are Digital Pathology Images "Captured"?

Basically, WSI hardware consists of a robotic/automated microscope with specialized acquisition software. Some instruments are more specialized and purpose-specific in their design and construction than others. The simplest setups consist of add-on cameras on top of conventional microscopes. This is a great start if all you

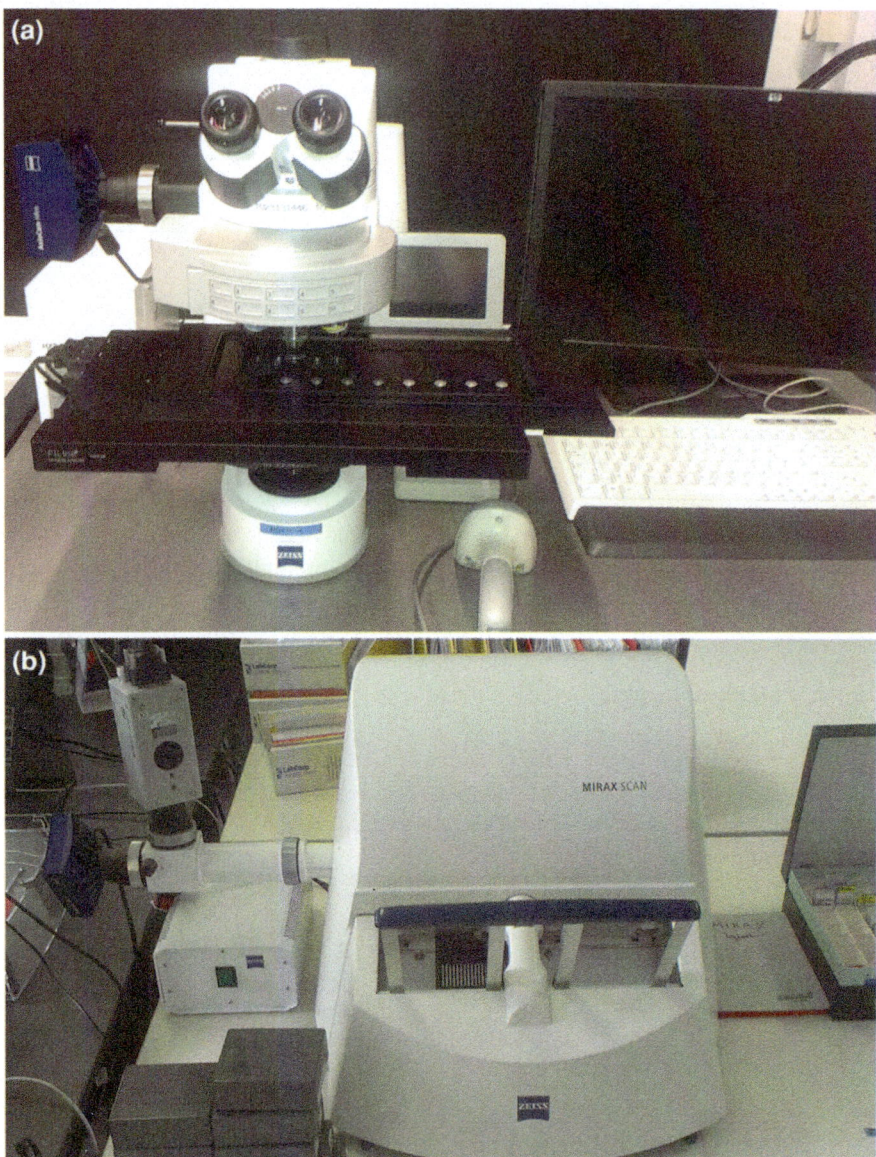

Fig. 2.1 a A Zeiss AxioVision setup with a mounted camera and robotic stage (courtesy of HistoGeneX). **b** A 3DHistech high-volume slide scanner (courtesy of HistoGeneX)

want to do is capture regions of interest (ROIs) and share them with colleagues or embed them in your publications. However, they are not necessarily suited for whole slide imaging. In order to do WSI, as well as systematically digitize your entire workflow, you need at least a robotic staging table as well. The robot then cooperates with the software component to move the slide, capturing individual

2.1 How Are Digital Pathology Images "Captured"?

ROIs that they are stitched back together to generate a WSI. Special viewing software is usually provided so that it appears that a seamless image was obtained by the entire slide. As an alternative, there also are devices like microscopes with mounted cameras but automated stages. The advantage is that viewed ROIs can be stored even when you switch between different slides (Fig. 2.1).

Technology has by now become sufficiently specialized so that some companies only sell complete integrated systems (scanners). However, others sell individual components as well. Examples of the latter are Hamamatsu, which sells its own Nanozoomer slide scanner as an integrated system, but also sells its components to TissueGnostics for their automated solutions.

2.2 How Do Slide Scanners Work?

Slide scanners are the highest level of abstraction for digital microscopy. They have both hardware and software components. We distinguish five levels, from lowest to highest: slide handling, slide scanning, optics, detection and, finally, acquisition software. These five levels are depicted in Fig. 2.2.

The first slide scanner was designed by James Bacus in 1994, during a period of rapid Internet expansion worldwide. The corresponding BLISS system, which is now recognized as having been the first virtual microscopy system ever developed, was designed to generate virtual microscope slides. Meanwhile, a WebSlide Server, Browser, and ActiveX Viewer were developed to allow for viewing virtual microscope slides over the Internet. Over the next several years, the Bacus Group developed and patented the methods and apparat to perform automated assays of biological specimens, immunoploidy analysis, measurements of tissue thickness, and tests of neoplasm progression, as well as devices to allow for the remote

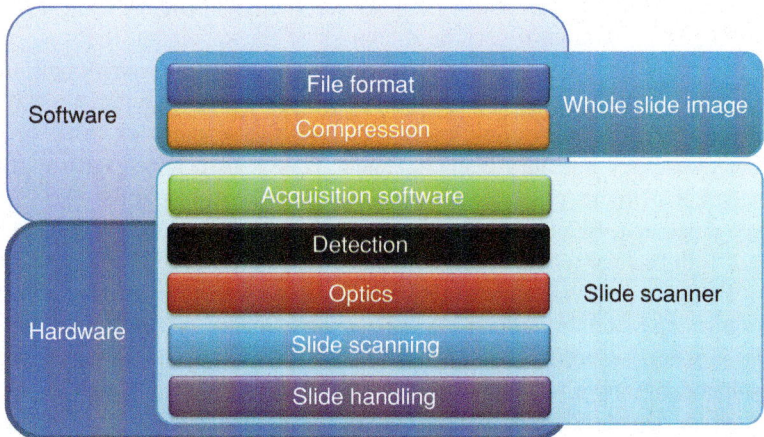

Fig. 2.2 Different layers of processing in digital pathology

control of microscopes, the creation of virtual microscopy slides, the magnification of specimen images, and the Internet, intranet, and local viewing of such slides [1–19]. Moreover, Bacus Laboratories not only created the first virtual slide system, and they also created the first market for it. They did this by framing their system as an educational tool. Their plan was to ultimately replace standard microscopes with virtual microscopy in medical education. They achieved this by combining their virtual microscopy system with a collection of educational "slides," for which institutions could lease access licenses annually. Because of its successful business model, Bacus Laboratories was purchased by Olympus America Inc. in 2006.

In terms of features, the capacities of slide scanners today vary widely. For example, some can do bright-field images only, some can do fluorescence images only, and some can do both. The price of a model generally correlates with its slide-loading capacity, which can range from one to 400 slides per batch. Slides can be handled as a single slide/stage, as stand-alone autoloaders ("hotels"), as slide trays, or as slide magazines. The type of slide can vary as well: While most scanners today still handle basic 1" × 3" slides only, others—such as Aperio and Huron Technologies—also support 2" × 3" and even larger (whole mount) slides. The more variability that is allowed for physical slide media, the harder it is to batch-process large numbers of slides.

Two approaches exist to scanning a slide: tile scanning (Bacus patents) [20] and line scanning (Aperio patents) [21]. In both cases, the resulting images (tiles or strips) are fitted together into a single large image (i.e., the WSI). With a tile scanner, the slide is scanned as a series of rectangular tiles. For each tile, the highest physical magnification desired is used (e.g., 40× or 20×). The tiles are then stacked into a WSI, like bricks forming a wall. This is done either concurrently with or after the scanning process, via the acquisition software. Conversely, with line scanning, after magnification, strips are combined side by side into a single image. Proponents of the latter approach claim that it generates fewer seams and, hence, fewer optical aberrations (Fig. 2.3).

One particular problem related to scanning is focusing. A pathologist looking through a microscope automatically adjusts the focus depending upon the area of the slide he or she is looking at, the thickness of the specimen, the type of glass slide used, etc. With a scanner, this process must be automated. With both tile and line scanners, it is possible to auto-focus each field after moving the stage, but this can be very time-consuming, especially with tile scanners. A better approach is to focus on every nth field being scanned. This is both faster and simpler; but the placement of focus points lacks context, and it is still possible to waste time on larger areas that, by chance, do not require refocusing. A focus map is another solution. With this approach, focus points are distributed over the tissue forming a surface. Focus is only recalculated for intervening tissue. The number of selected focus points can be controlled via the scanner software. A trade-off is usually made between more focus points (less speed) and greater accuracy. The settings can be tissue-dependent, and a technician can maintain a preset list of "profiles" that can be referred to, depending upon the type of specimen that needs to be scanned.

Z-stacking is becoming increasingly commonplace, but this poses its own unique challenges to file format organization (see later in this chapter). The new frontier is now spectral imaging.

2.3 Virtual Slide Formats

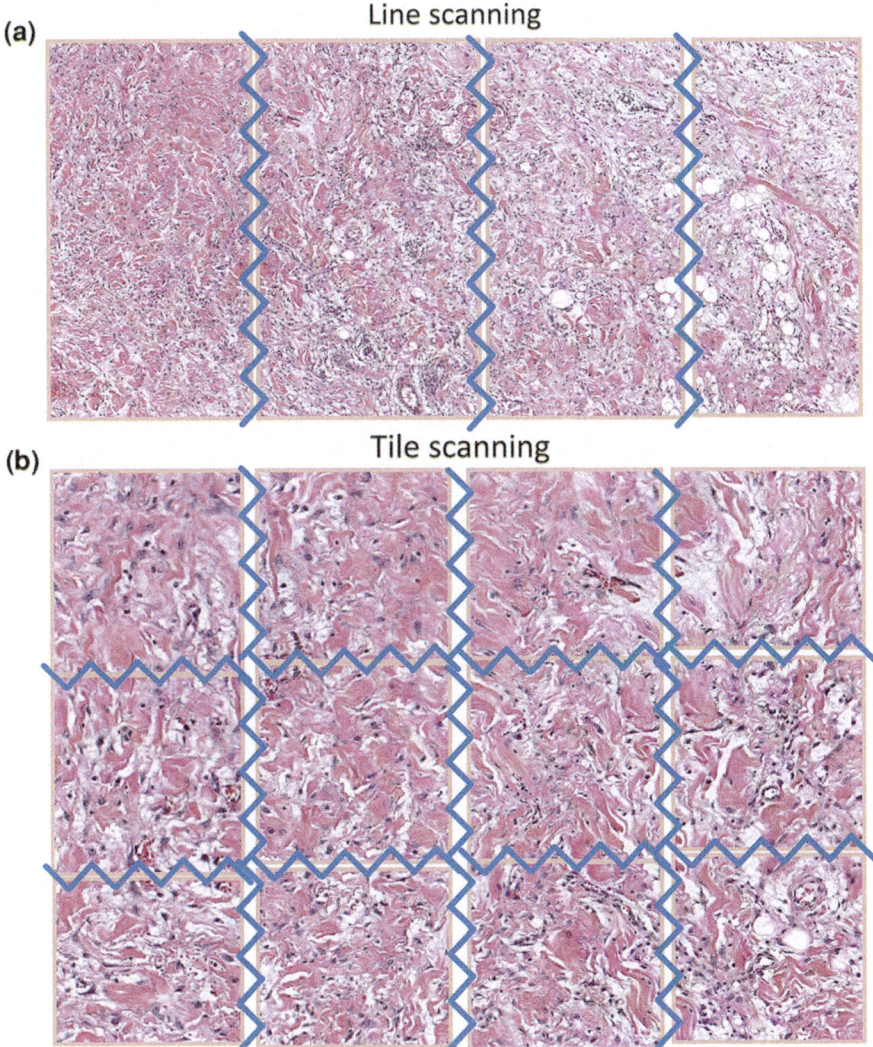

Fig. 2.3 a/b Tile versus line scanning: note the huge decrease in the number of seams with line scanning

2.3 Virtual Slide Formats

2.3.1 How Are WSI Data Organized?

After the acquisition software in the scanner obtains a digital image representation of a slide, it needs to store this information somewhere. This again can be seen as a two-step process, whereby first data compression takes place and subsequently data are stored, usually in a vendor-specific file format.

Digital slide image formats typically consist of one or more files that contain high-resolution scanned areas as well as image information in the form of metadata. The resolution of such images varies, but usually ranges from ten to hundreds of thousands of pixels per dimension (width and height). Various techniques are currently employed to make it easier and quicker to process such images using computer software.

2.3.2 The Pyramidal Format

Scaled versions of the original image (called "zoom levels") are often created and stored in a single "container" format. This is usually called a "pyramidal format," since every scaled-down image is smaller than its previous level, just like a pyramid gets smaller and smaller the higher up you go. By storing pre-computed scaled-down versions of the high-resolution image, a computer program can quickly render a smaller version of the image by reading pixel data from the zoom level closest to the scale currently being displayed.

The pyramidal format increases display performance at the cost of storage efficiency. For this reason, many vendors try to minimize the actual scan area that is being stored. This is done by spotting the significant areas while scanning the slide and only storing these in high resolution. This leads to a digital slide image with many sparse high-resolution areas, which may follow the pyramidal format independently. For different tissue types, the tissue detection parameters (called "profiles" by some vendors) often must be fine-tuned (Fig. 2.4).

2.3.3 Tiles

To further optimize random access and minimize disk read operations (input/output or I/O), digital slides split the image into smaller rectangular areas (tiles). Every zoom level is therefore a grid of tiles of the same size. When a computer program needs to display a small part of a high-resolution image, it is able to reduce the data being read by selecting only those tiles that intersect with the current viewport.

Slide scanning is performed in steps. The scanner's camera moves along the slide and takes pictures which are then stitched together by the scanner's software. Some vendors decide to store overlapping images of the slide and let the viewing software do the stitching. This is done because selecting stitching offsets that depend on the visible parts of the image every time may reduce stitching artifacts. This, in turn, would have otherwise been introduced if stitching had happened during scanning. In this case, stitching hints are stored as metadata along with the image.

Regardless of when the stitching process takes place (during scanning or while the image is viewed), images acquired by the scanner require adjustments. Overlapping regions might have differences in brightness and contrast, known as *shading*, due to the different positions of the camera, each time a photograph is taken. Various techniques are employed to address this issue, such as blending and histogram equalization.

2.4 Vendor-Specific File Format Implementations

2.4.1 TIFF-based Formats

2.4.1.1 TIFF

TIFF images are used by scanner vendors to store digital slides. The TIFF format natively supports storing images in grids of tiles and is generally well suited for random access. It allows for multiple images (directories) to be stored within a single file and for various compression schemes to be used. Since a slide's size may overcome the maximum 4-GB threshold, the BigTIFF format is also common. It essentially uses 64-bit pointers to store offsets within the file.

Typically, one tiled TIFF directory is the high-resolution image, while several others may follow that are down-scaled versions of the original. One downside of the plain TIFF format is that there is no definitive way to specify which directory is for the high-resolution image and which are for the down-scaled images, because the specifications do not anticipate relationships between the directories. The display software attempts to overcome this by making assumptions; for example, the largest directory (in width or height) may be considered the original image and every other directory a smaller zoom level.

2.4.1.2 Open Microscopy Environment (OME) TIFF (Extensions .tif, .tiff)

The OME-TIFF format was designed to incorporate both the rich metadata that is included within the OME-XML format, and the pixels that exist within the multi-page TIFF format. In this way, it is compatible with a much broader range of applications. There are several other main features of OME-TIFF datasets that make them distinct from other formats [22].

First, each and every dataset contains image planes that are stored either within a single multi-page TIFF file, or spanning multiple TIFF files. With either of these options, virtually any image organization scheme is possible.

Second, embedded within each TIFF file's header there is a complete OME-XML metadata block that describes the dataset. In this way, the metadata remain intact even if some of the dataset's TIFF files become displaced. This OME-XML metadata block can contain anything that is permitted within a standard OME-XML file.

Third, the standard TIFF mechanism is used to store one or more image planes in each of the constituent files, rather than encoding pixels as Base64 chunks within the XML. Since TIFF is an image format, when there is at least one image plane, it makes sense to use OME-TIFF instead of OME-XML.

A more complete description of the OME-TIFF format, including companies that support it, public image repositories that permit image downloads as OME-TIFF, more detailed technical information, an example code, and sample data, is available online at https://www.openmicroscopy.org/site/support/ome-model/ome-tiff/.

2.4.1.3 Ventana BIF (Extension .bif)

Ventana slides are stored in single-file BigTIFF format. The first directory contains a label image, usually in tiled format. The label image is a thumbnail that includes the actual physical label for the glass slide. The directory specifies the XMP tag (700) and stores valid XML metadata about the slide. Next comes a thumbnail, and the high-resolution image follows.

BIF images contain overlapping tiles, for which an appropriate algorithm is required for them to be correctly rendered. The directory containing the high-resolution images also specifies the XMP tag that contains tile stitching hints between neighboring tiles. The rendering algorithm calculates global coordinates for every tile, based upon these hints. This may result in stitching artifacts in parts of the image. Subsequent image directories do not have such information, and tile positions are calculated via reduction to the base level.

2.4.1.4 Other TIFF Formats

Several other vendors use derivatives of the TIFF format. These include Leica SCN, Aperio SVS, Trestle, and Hamamatsu NDPI. Sometimes, it suffices to rename the proprietary file extension into .tif to visualize files in common software packages such as Adobe Photoshop. Several file formats are then documented in more detail at the OpenSlide project: http://www.openslide.org/formats.

2.4.2 Other Format Types

Not all vendors follow the TIFF format. 3DHISTECH Mirax (.mrxs extension) slides are stored in a multi-file JPEG format with proprietary metadata and indexes. One slide corresponds to many files in a single folder. Each file contains an aspect of the format, such as an overview image, a particular zoom level, or annotation data. The index files information on where to find particular pieces of data into the individual .dat files.

The Olympus file format (.vsi extension) is derived from TIFF. Like Mirax, it consists of a collection of different files in a single folder, with the .vsi file serving as an index file. Olympus files can contain multiple regions of the same physical slide, scanned at variable levels of resolution. High-resolution pixel data are stored in extensible tile server (.ets) files that are maintained in subdirectories (defined in the "main" .vsi file). ETS is a proprietary file format that is used to store multi-dimensional data organized in tiles. In most instances, a single region of a slide is stored in tiled pyramidal fashion within an ETS file.

Finally, there is Zeiss. Like Hamamatsu and Leica, Zeiss has multiple file formats defined for whole slide imaging. The CZI format was designed to mimic open microscopy environment (OME) specifications (http://www.openmicroscopy.org).

2.4 Vendor-Specific File Format Implementations

It is intended to be maximally compatible with OME-TIFF and OME-XML data formats, while maintaining the specifications that are essential to optimize the use of Carl Zeiss ZEN software.

ZVI is older than the CZI format, but still widely because of the widespread use of the platforms that use it. AxioVision is one of the programs that support the format, and a plug-in for ImageJ is also available (and comes standard with the Fiji toolbox). Within a ZVI file, a multi-dimensional space is defined to facilitate time-lapse, multiple (fluorescent) channels, and mosaic-style recordings.

Additional information on each format can be found here (sometimes after signing a license agreement):

- Mirax—http://openslide.org/formats/mirax/
- Olympus—http://cbis.nus.edu.sg/wp-content/uploads/2012/05/Manual_cellSens_en.pdf
- Zeiss CZI—http://www.zeiss.com/microscopy/en_de/downloads/zen.html
- Zeiss ZVI—http://applications.zeiss.com/c1257a26004b6e67/allbysubject/7824899fee4f1290c1257c050044fb18

2.4.3 The Role of DICOM

As the proverbial 800-pound gorilla in the room, DICOM deserves its own paragraph. DICOM stands for Digital Imaging and Communication in Medicine and is a network maintained by the National Electronic Manufacturer's Association (NEMA) and supported by large-image management systems called picture archive and communication systems (PACS). Various PACS systems are used in hospitals and laboratories to manage images used for clinical and research purposes in medicine; this includes, among other functions, their storage, and retrieval.

Since 2009, a new supplement has been added to the DICOM standard. This supplement is known as "Supp 145, Whole Slide Imaging in Pathology." The supplement was developed by Workgroup 26 and describes how an extension has been made to the DICOM standard to allow for the storage of very large images. The DICOM standard defines a family set for the image, called "instances" as per the DICOM vocabulary. All these instances follow an information object definition which is defined in PS 3.3; currently, version 2011 is the latest available. In all those IODs, DICOM instances have columns and rows defined as unsigned short values. What this means is that, in theory, all images must be 64K columns and rows. WSI frequently have images much larger than these pixel dimensions.

Rather than follow what occurs during the TIFF to BigTIFF (64-bit extension) transition, the DICOM committee chose a different, very conservative approach, whereby the unsigned short value for the column and row does not change. Instead, new attributes are added to store the actual pixel dimension. In this scenario, a single WSI cannot be stored within a single "instance." Instead, a single WSI is inserted in fragments at a series level.

The proposed approach guarantees that all legacy software remains able to process any incoming WSI series, since the attributes in columns and rows are still defined as unsigned short.

One should notice, though, that this supplement pushes the DICOM standard to the edge, since uncompressed pixel data stored within a single DICOM instance are limited to a 232 − 1 byte (4 GB minus a byte, 0xFFFFFFFF being a reserved value). Therefore, the lower level of this pyramid is unlikely to be saved in uncompressed form, since its total size will likely exceed that limit considerably. In such a case, it is assumed that another transfer syntax will be used for those larger pyramid levels (e.g., JPEG). When using an encapsulated transfer syntax (e.g., JPEG type), there is no such limit, and all individual tiles can be stored within a single DICOM instance.

2.5 Do-It-Yourself Programming

For people who have experience with programming (be it in a full-blown framework like Java or a scripting language like Python), options exist to get right to work interacting with the data from the various hardware vendors.

OpenSlide is written in C, having its origins at Carnegie Mellon University (93;94). It has binary distributions for various flavors of the Linux operating system, as well as for Windows. Individuals have also reported on how to deploy the library on Apple hardware. Instructions on how to deploy the software on each of the respective platforms are provided on their Web site http://www.openslide.org.

An alternative library is the BioFormats project. This was initially developed at the University of Wisconsin–Madison [23]. BioFormats is written in Java and has a wider selection of supported file formats, but some currently used microscopy formats are missing or only partially implemented. Extensive documentation on the library is provided through the OpenMicroscopy portal at http://www.openmicroscopy.org.

The goals of OpenSlide and BioFormats are slightly different. While both can be used to read proprietary vendor formats, OpenSlide was started as a project to visualize large images. Meanwhile, BioFormats is seen as a way to convert a proprietary format into an intermediate format (OME-TIFF, cf. supra). Perhaps this also explains why OpenSlide seems more performant than BioFormats; it is unlikely that one would do this conversion in real time.

If workflow permits it, BioFormats can simplify matters, because a single file format is the outcome (although OpenSlide abstracts things as well). The file format furthermore not only has image data, but capabilities for additional annotation, something that OpenSlide deliberately avoids.

If you decide that you want to process your own WSI data, you should consider the file format that you work with. OpenSlide is the only one that supports 3DHistech's MRXS format, whereas BioFormats is the only one that (at least partially) supports the Olympus and Zeiss formats.

2.6 Bits, Bytes, and Wires

This book is not intended as guidelines on how you can build your own scanner or write your own WSI viewer software. Nevertheless, no review of digital pathology can be complete without also addressing the hardware and software involved. We have tried to introduce you to some of the intricacies of engineering that were required to develop slide scanners in the first place. Then, we moved on to the software side of things: How are WSI data stored? This is something that we all get exposed to, if only by transferring slides to a colleague via a USB memory key.

Slide scanners have not been around all that long. Two basic modes of operation exist for scanners, and virtually all scanners on the market today can be traced back to one or two sets of patents. Data captured by the slide scanner must be stored on the hard disk of the user's computer and organized so that it can be visualized optimally. File formats have been devised by different vendors to accomplish this. Because of the pixel size of the raw data (roughly 1,500 times more than the digital camera that you use on vacation) and the different features of the scanners (bright-field, fluorescence, confocal, etc.), various solutions have been thought of. However, these differences make it hard to move from one digital pathology platform to another, and one risks vendor lock-in because of this. Some initiatives for standardization have already been undertaken and are expected to become more center stage in the future.

References

1. Bacus, J.V., Bacus, J.W.: Method and apparatus for processing an image of a tissue sample microarray. US Patent 6,466,690 (2000). Ref type: Patent
2. Bacus, J.V., Bacus, J.W.: Method and apparatus for acquiring and reconstructing magnified specimen images from a computer-controlled microscope. US Patent 6,101,265 (2000). Ref type: Patent
3. Bacus, J.V., Bacus, J.W.: Method and apparatus for acquiring and reconstructing magnified specimen images from a computer-controlled microscope. US Patent 6,226,392 (2001). Ref type: Patent
4. Bacus, J.V., Bacus, J.W.: Method and apparatus for creating a virtual microscope slide. US Patent 6,272,235 (2001). Ref type: Patent
5. Bacus, J.V., Bacus, J.W.: Method and apparatus for acquiring and reconstructing magnified specimen images from a computer-controlled microscope. US Patent 6,404,906 (2002). Ref type: Patent
6. Bacus, J.V., Bacus, J.W.: Apparatus for remote control of a microscope. US Patent 6,674,884 (2004). Ref type: Patent
7. Bacus, J.V., Bacus, J.W.: Method and apparatus for creating a virtual microscope slide. US Patent 6,775,402 (2004). Ref type: Patent
8. Bacus, J.V., Bacus, J.W.: Apparatus for remote control of a microscope. US Patent 7,110,586 (2006). Ref type: Patent
9. Bacus, J.V., Bacus, J.W.: Method and apparatus for creating a virtual microscope slide. US Patent 7,146,372 (2006). Ref type: Patent
10. Bacus, J.V., Bacus, J.W.: Method and apparatus for internet, intranet, and local viewing of virtual microscope slides. US Patent 7,149,332 (2006). Ref type: Patent

11. Bacus, J.W., Bacus, J.V.: Method and apparatus for automated assay of biological specimens. US Patent 5,473,706 (1995). Ref type: Patent
12. Bacus, J.W.: Method and apparatus for automated analysis of biological specimens. US Patent 5,526,258 (1996). Ref type: Patent
13. Bacus, J.W., Marder, J.M.: Method and apparatus for immunoploidy analysis. US Patent 5,541,064 (1996). Ref type: Patent
14. Bacus, J.W., Bacus, J.V.: Method and apparatus for measuring tissue section thickness. US Patent 5,546,323 (1996). Ref type: Patent
15. Bacus, J.W., Oud, P.S.: Apparatus and method for analysis of biological specimens. US Patent 5,485,527 (1996). Ref type: Patent
16. Bacus, J.W., Bacus, J.V.: Method and apparatus for testing a progression of neoplasia including cancer chemoprevention testing. US Patent 6,031,930 (2000). Ref type: Patent
17. Bacus, J.W., Bacus, J.V.: Method and apparatus for internet, intranet, and local viewing of virtual microscope slides. US Patent 6,396,941 (2002). Ref type: Patent
18. Bacus, J.W., Bacus, J.V.: Method and apparatus for creating a virtual microscope slide. US Patent 6,522,774 (2003). Ref type: Patent
19. Bacus, J.W., Bacus, J.V.: Method and apparatus for internet, intranet, and local viewing of virtual microscope slides. US Patent 6,674,881 (2004). Ref type: Patent
20. James W.: Bacus patents. JamesBacus.com. (2014). Ref type: Electronic Citation
21. Aperio Technologies Inc., Patent Applications. Patentdocs. (2014). Ref type: Electronic Citation
22. El Saghir, N.S., Keating, N.L., Carlson, R.W., Khoury, K.E., Fallowfield, L.: Tumor boards: optimizing the structure and improving efficiency of multidisciplinary management of patients with cancer worldwide. Am. Soc. Clin. Oncol. Educ. Book **34**, e461–e466 (2014)
23. Marshall, C.L., Petersen, N.J., Naik, A.D., et al.: Implementation of a regional virtual tumor board: a prospective study evaluating feasibility and provider acceptance. Telemed. J. E. Health (20 May 2014) (Epub ahead of print)

About the Authors

Dr. Sucaet and Dr. Waelput are co-founders of Pathomation, a young but rapidly-growing company that offers a range of novel but proven software products and solutions to manage and share digital pathology data.

Since its inception as the result of an internal software development project that commenced in 2011, Pathomation has been developing digital pathology software for healthcare and life science environments. The company born out of a very real need that was observed by its co-founders when they both worked at HistoGeneX. Central to its product offers is a vendor-agnostic image server, which recognizes DP-specific file formats, including SCN, MRXS, NDPI, TIFF, SVS, ZVI, VMS and VMU. The PathoCore data server sits as a broker between the company's different visualization and data transfer modules. The company also offers digital pathology-specific slide viewers that target the client's desktop, intranet/internet environment, or the public cloud, as needed. In addition to viewers, it has developed plug-ins for different popular image processing software programs, like PhotoShop and ImageJ.

The company's core beliefs are (1) that versatility is key (since different organ systems require different evaluation methods and modalities); but also (2) that control and supervision are even more important, given increasing regulatory requirements. Its commitment to clients is to surpass all expectations on both beliefs.

To find out more about Pathomation's many products and services, visit http://www.pathomation.com.

Index

B
BIF, 25
Biobank, 35, 37
Biomarker, 57–59, 68

D
3D imaging, 73
Digital pathology (DP), 1, 2, 4–10, 15, 17, 22, 27, 28, 31–35, 37–39, 48–50, 61, 62, 64–68, 71–73, 75–78
Digital pathology application, 68, 75, 78
Digital pathology future, 77
Digital pathology history, 1

F
File format, 19, 22, 26, 28

H
Histological analysis, 44, 46, 47

I
Image analysis, 44, 45, 48, 50
Informatics, 4, 6

L
Line scanner, 18

M
Medical imaging, 27
Medical systems biology, 72, 78
Micro-CT, 71
MRXS, 25

N
NDPI, 25

O
Object recognition, 50

P
Pathology applications, 31
Pathology cockpit, 6
Pathology dashboard, 6
Pathology education, 31
Primary diagnosis, 38, 39, 66, 68

Q
Quality assurance, 32, 33, 36, 37, 65, 67, 68

S
Second opinion, 33, 40, 64, 65, 68
Slide scanner, 17, 18, 22, 28
Spectral imaging, 74
SVS, 24

T
Telepathology, 1, 2, 4–6, 8, 9, 57, 60, 64, 65
Third World, 76
Tile scanner, 18
Tumor board, 31, 34

W
Whole slide imaging (WSI), 5, 6, 8–10, 15, 20, 22, 27, 58, 60–62, 64

The manufacturer's authorised representative in the EU is Springer Nature Customer Service Centre GmbH, Europaplatz 3, 69115 Heidelberg, Germany. If you have any concerns regarding our products, please contact ProductSafety@springernature.com

Printed and bound by CPI Group (UK) Ltd, Croydon, CR0 4YY

23/03/2026

02076369-0003